The Myth of
Neuropsychiatry

A Look at
Paradoxes, Physics,
and the Human Brain

The Myth of Neuropsychiatry

A Look at Paradoxes, Physics, and the Human Brain

Donald Mender, M. D.

Plenum Press • New York and London

Library of Congress Cataloging in Publication Data

Mender, Donald.
  The myth of neuropsychiatry: a look at paradoxes, physics, and the human brain
/ Donald Mender.
     p.   cm.
  Includes bibliographical references and index.
  ISBN 0-306-44652-9
  1. Neuropsychiatry—Philosophy. 2. Psychiatry—Philosophy. 3. Mind-brain
identity theory. I. Title.
  [DNLM: 1. Mental Disorders. 2. Brain Diseases—physiopathology. WM 100
M5375m 1994]
RC343.M44   1994
616.8—dc20
DNLM/DLC   94-2840
for Library of Congress   CIP

ISBN 0-306-44652-9

© 1994 Donald Mender
Plenum Press is a Division of Plenum Publishing Corporation
233 Spring Street, New York, N.Y. 10013-1578

Printed in the United States of America

Contents

1

The Rise of Modern Neuropsychiatry

A psychiatrist, sitting in his office today, faces an awesome array of challenges. He has to deal with government bureaucracies, malpractice insurance, competing professionals, and the need for continuing education. A beeper and answering service constantly test his mettle. But most importantly, he has to decide among a bewildering host of options in his approach to each individual patient.

For example, a typical practitioner may look out into his waiting room one day to find an unfamiliar, elderly, disheveled woman sent by a colleague for evaluation. She may mutter to herself, shuffle, ignore her surroundings, finally slump into a chair, and not bother even to leaf through magazines on the coffee table. Inside the doctor's consulting room, the woman may have trouble mustering enough energy to answer questions about her symptoms. She may apologize inappropriately for taking up the doctor's time, or begin to cry.

The psychiatrist who encounters such a patient will know immediately that depression is a likely diagnosis. He will make sure to get enough information about the patient to assess any risk of suicide and rule out other conditions. But then the doctor's next step will be the formulation of a treatment plan. Here he will have to choose from a number of alternatives.

As a psychotherapist, he might elect to have his patient return for frequent counseling sessions that address feelings of loss, guilt, and hidden anger. He might target self-defeating behavior as a focus for change. He might prescribe antidepressant drugs or even electroshock. Or he might arrange admission to a hospital for medical tests.

How does a psychiatrist make these kinds of choices? As an independent agent, of course, he follows his own judgment and tailors treatment to the particular needs of each person in his care. But as a member of a larger psychiatric community, he may be influenced by fashions and trends.

ﰿ   ﰿ   ﰿ

Anyone who wants to discover currents in thinking among doctors will do well to sample articles in the medical profession's top periodicals.

Some of the most telling and influential statements by leading physicians appear in the prestigious *New England Journal of Medicine*, especially through its "Special Articles." In 1979, this series became a forum for the views of a particularly famous and thoughtful medical scientist, Eric Kandel.

Dr. Kandel is now University Professor at Columbia College of Physicians and Surgeons and Senior Investigator at the Howard Hughes Institute. He was born in Vienna and emigrated to America in 1939. He attended Harvard College and New York University School of Medicine, interned at Montefiore Hospital in New York City, and was a psychiatric resident at the Massachusetts Mental Health Center. His laboratory research career began at the National Institute of Mental Health in suburban Maryland and at the Institute Marey in Paris, where collaboration with Ladislav Tauc led to his important work in basic neuroscience. He joined the faculty of NYU in 1965.[1]

Dr. Kandel's unusually diverse background as a clinically

trained psychiatrist also skilled in the study of single nerve cells helped him open mental phenomena to the scrutiny of laboratory scientists. His team of investigators sought and found mechanisms for simple learning processes in the nervous tissue of primitive creatures like snails. Dr. Kandel's efforts were recognized by his peers, and he became an important voice among behavioral neurobiologists. By the time his article appeared in the *New England Journal*, he had established himself at Columbia as a highly regarded faculty member, directing its Division of Neurobiology and Behavior.[2]

Dr. Kandel's Special Article was published on November 8, 1979. He called it "Psychotherapy and the Single Synapse: The Impact of Psychiatric Thought on Neurobiologic Research." It had been adapted from a lecture that he had given eighteen months earlier at the Harvard Club in Boston. Its prescient contents summarized the consequences of a developing revolution that continues in full force today. That revolution is called neuropsychiatry.

Dr. Kandel began his article by describing a schism that he had noticed among his fellow psychiatrists during residency training. His colleagues had separated into two groups: "soft-nosed" Freudian psychotherapists and those who wanted a more exact, "hard-nosed," biological approach to mental disorders. Many of the latter hoped that a basis for precision in psychiatry might emerge from studies of the brain.[3,4]

Dr. Kandel went on to show that this schism had influenced the psychiatric profession at large. He suggested the possibility of a conceptual bridge between the two warring camps, linking "hard-nosed" and "soft-nosed" views more harmoniously. In a subtle discussion, he used the views of a famed sociobiologist, Edward O. Wilson, to describe the neuroscientific community's relationship to analytic psychiatry. Dr. Kandel suggested that Freudian approaches to psychology, while " potentially deeper in content" than neurobiology, could profit from recent technical advances that promised to endow brain laboratories with great exploratory power. Analytic psychologists and psychiatrists could now set agendas and ask questions about neurological mechanisms in mental health and illness; neuroscientists armed with new research tools could cooperate by providing answers.[5]

Dr. Kandel illustrated his point with emerging ideas about the neurobiology of learning and psychological growth in childhood. He cited the work of Rene Spitz, Harry Harlow, Austin Riesen, David Hubel, and Torsen Wiesel to show how emotional damage to infants who had been deprived of contact with their mothers might involve brain mechanisms. He also drew on his own important work.

During the course of his discussion, Dr. Kandel was careful to caution readers that the link between properties of brain tissue and mental attributes is not simple.[6] However, since the *New England Journal* article first appeared, other psychiatrists have increasingly moved toward extreme neurological approaches to mental illness. Many have become firm believers in the total reduction of psychiatry to "hard-nosed" neuroscience. Prominent academic leaders have declared that the future of psychiatry hinges not on psychology at all, but only on biology. They have argued that the psyche is only a metaphor for the way our brain works, that mental aberrations merely represent disorders of its physiology, and that psychiatry should therefore focus its energies on medical treatments for the illnesses under its purview.

The main ideas of these "hard-nosed" neuropsychiatrists might be summarized as follows:

1. The mind exists primarily as a by-product of brain activity.
2. Mental aberrations arise from disturbed brain function.
3. Analysis of physical brain events, not disembodied thought processes, offers the best route to diagnosis of psychiatric illness.
4. Effective treatment of psychiatric maladies works by modifying abnormal brain functions.

These views, which are gaining a wider and wider hearing, clearly fly in the face of the more "soft-nosed" among Freudian psychoanalysts. They also run in strong opposition to the opinions of many other therapeutic schools. Not all these groups rely on the couch to treat mental disorders. But every one of them has at least a faction that embraces abstract concepts of the mind with no anchor in the physical world. It is that disembodiment that "hard-nosed" neuropsychiatry is out to demolish.

        🙜   🙜   🙜

No one can really blame a psychiatrist for going out on a conceptual limb in search of solutions to the problem of mental illness. Whether his professional outlook embraces the neo-Freudian movements that dominated America in the 1950s, the community mental health programs of the activist 1960s, or current biological trends, a psychiatrist must witness suffering that begs for relief.

The most painful aspects of human existence have always centered around passions out of control. Authors from the time of Euripides onward have dealt with the impact of emotional storms on our lives. Sophocles' ancient Greek play *Oedipus Tyrranus*, 2300 years after its first production, became the nucleus of Freudian psychology. The concern that every person feels about his darker nature has resurfaced again and again throughout history.

All kinds of people suffer from infirmities of the mind. Some of the most famous have included Joan of Arc, Abraham Lincoln, and Vincent van Gogh. Records of physicians encountering psychiatric disorders have come down to us from ancient India, Israel, Egypt, Greece, and Rome. Phenomena that medieval culture regarded as satanic possession probably grew out of mental illness.[7,8]

Some psychiatric diseases have remained unchanged across the boundaries of time and place. Schizophrenia, for example, has always stood as the prototype of madness. Although labels and definitions have varied slightly, a core of psychotic symptoms and signs always seems to affect its victims. These characteristics include odd patterns of thinking, avoidance of other people, strange or deadpan facial expressions, and decay of the personality with advancing age. Delusions and hallucinations also add to the mental havoc of the disorder. Many who suffer from schizophrenia end up living on the street or in government asylums, cut off from everything that makes normal life worth living. A typical schizophrenic case history in modern America might run as follows:

According to his parents, Robert R. had always been a loner, but no one ever thought him mentally disturbed until he left home for college. He couldn't adapt to dormitory life or to the social scene. His assigned roommate, an amateur guitarist, complained that Robert objected to music of any kind and especially hated the electronic sounds that came from a stereo system down the hall. Robert began to spend long hours in the bathroom rather than join bridge games, bull sessions, or forays with other students to the campus watering hole. He didn't seem interested in girls or platonic friendships. His grades held up at first, but even the academic part of his life began to fall apart after three months at school.

On the night before his first final examination, Robert appeared, half-naked and drenched with sweat, in the room housing the stereo system that he disliked. He threatened its owner with a "curse" unless the equipment was destroyed. The campus police were called; they arrived shortly and took Robert to a local emergency room.

A psychiatrist there questioned him. He discovered Robert's long-held belief that dials on the stereo amplifier had tuned into his brain as part of a worldwide plot to control his thoughts. Robert actually claimed to hear voice transmissions from the headquarters of this conspiracy. He blamed the stereo system for his social and academic failure in college, but seemed peculiarly bland while talking about this upsetting matter. Blood tests, taken when he arrived at the emergency ward, showed no medical condition or street drugs to account for his strange state of mind. It was decided to admit him to the hospital.

Ten years later, the same psychiatrist who had first encountered Robert ran across him again. He had never returned to college and was now a chronic patient in a large municipal clinic. His days were spent, unemployed and friendless, wandering subways and city parks in a dirty pair of overalls. A variety of treatments had prevented blowups that might return him to the hospital, but no measures existed that could prevent the long-term decline into his present situation.

Schizophrenia differs from another mental disturbance called manic–depressive illness.[9] Persons burdened with this second infirmity exhibit wild swings in mood. On some days, such patients launch into frenzied peaks of energy, producing endless chatter, physical overactivity, grandiose beliefs, and bizarre lapses in judgment. At other times, the same patients descend into the depths of despair, torture themselves with guilt, and lose even the desire to eat or sleep. In some cases victims experience only one kind of mood swing, either manic excitement or depressive melancholia, without ever flipping into the other emotional state. Between attacks of illness, behavior returns to normal, unlike the situation in schizophrenia. But the threat of death by exhaustion or suicide for manic–depressive patients always lurks in the future. A case illustrating such features might evolve in the following manner:

> A 37-year-old Chicago attorney named Kathy N. found one day that she was on a roll. Her briefs seemed easier and easier to write; she didn't even need references from the law library to turn out a first-class product. Finished papers flew out of her typewriter almost faster than she could feed blank sheets into the carriage.
>
> Kathy soon decided that the Supreme Court needed her services. She rushed to the bank, emptied her savings

account, hailed a cab, and directed it toward the airport. To celebrate her departure for Washington, Kathy gave the taxi driver a $2000 tip. Finally, at an airline ticket counter, she realized that she was shouting incoherently at a clerk. He asked her to step aside and called a security guard, who escorted Kathy to a private waiting area. Forty minutes later, she found herself in a downtown psychiatric ward.

After several weeks, Kathy recovered enough of her own senses to understand that she had suffered her third manic spell. During her first, at the age of 20, she had to be stopped by friends from bicycling across a rising drawbridge. After the second, she had accepted the need for psychiatric care. Now she only hoped that her finances had survived the third attack. Despite her lavish tip for the cab driver, it turned out that the rest of her funds were safe.

One week later, Kathy began to grow despondent over her $2000 loss. Her thoughts became more and more exclusively preoccupied with the wasted money. She came to believe falsely that all her assets had been bled dry, that creditors would soon knock on her door, and that she deserved no less because of her foolish profligacy. She stopped sleeping or eating and began to think about ending it all. The hospital staff promptly started antidepressant treatment.

A long list of additional psychiatric maladies may be added to the schizophrenic and manic–depressive syndromes described above. Among the "dissociative" disturbances, for example, hysteria—a combination of seductive behavior and elusive physical symptoms—has perplexed physicians for centuries and piqued the interest of medical giants as far back as Hippocrates. Criminal personality disorders have greatly occupied the keepers of public order in every human society since recorded history began. More recently, attention has turned to yet other mental illnesses, sometimes called neuroses or anxiety states. Obsessive–compulsive syndromes are among the most disabling of these; affected patients are locked into magic rituals intended to ward off recurrent anxiety. Phobias cripple victims by burdening them with stubborn and unrealistic fears that inhibit the activities of normal living. Panic disorders flood otherwise calm individuals with inexplicable spasms of terror and the expectation of death.

Together, all these mental afflictions continue to cause untold misery even in our enlightened society. They pervade human experience and appear in all sorts of environments. At least one in 10 people suffers from depression. Up to one in 13 must endure anxiety attacks. One in 100 develops schizophrenia.[10]

Lives are often disrupted or ended. Nine of every ten people who kill themselves carry the burden of a psychiatric diagnosis. Half of all suicides have a history of depression. One tenth of the patients afflicted with schizophrenia die by their own hand.[11,12]

Families and even whole communities are harmed. Most of the damage is subtle, but some people in the midst of manic episodes, schizophrenic decline, or antisocial activities act with outright violence toward others.[13,14] Depressive, antisocial, and schizophrenic symptoms drive a number of sufferers each year to abuse drugs.[15] Americans have had to erect a costly forensic system to help process such consequences through the courts.

        è   è   è

The biological viewpoint that has burgeoned among psychiatrists in recent decades to explain and cope with these destructive problems is not without its historical precedents. For example, ancient physicians trying to find relief for their patients speculated about causes of mental illness that were rooted in the body rather than the mind. The two most prominent such healers were Hippocrates and Galen.

Hippocrates was born about 460 BC on the island of Cos. He worked as a physician throughout Greece until returning home to found a school of followers. His writings and those of his disciples fill over 70 notebooks, which provide evidence that he invented the modern practice of recording case histories. Hippocrates also codified his ideas on medical ethics in the Hippocratic Oath, still sworn by physicians today. He died in about 380 BC.[16]

Hippocrates believed that wanderings of the uterus through the bodies of hysterical women caused their behavioral difficulties. He also taught that psychological disturbances come from the effect on the brain of imbalanced bodily fluids or "humors." Hippocrates designated these humors as black bile, phlegm, yellow bile, and blood; they derived from the four basic elements, earth, air, fire, and water, and the two basic qualities, heat and moisture, all of which earlier Greeks had posited as the ground of existence. According to Hippocrates and his successors, each humor embodies a unique combination of gradations in heat and moisture. Blood is ostensibly warm and moist, phlegm cold and moist, yellow bile hot and dry, and black bile cold and dry.

Through Galen, such views eventually grew into a doctrine that humors create all human temperaments. Galen lived in the second century AD, studied medicine in Greece, and ministered to powerful Romans like Commodus, Sextus, Severus, and the emperor Marcus Aurelius.[17,18] Galen promoted the idea that yellow bile or choler produces quick-tempered behavior, blood a "sanguine" style, phlegm a cool or apathetic manner, and black bile "melancholia." He thus explained mental illness by blaming, for example, abnormal memory loss on a buildup of phlegm and pathologically destructive behavior on an excess of yellow bile. Galen's concepts came to dominate European medicine for centuries.[19–22]

During the European Middle Ages, a Frenchman, Bartholomaeus Anglicus, hinted at a neuropsychiatric viewpoint by trying to connect specific psychological traits, both normal and abnormal, with particular parts of the central nervous system. Four hundred years later in England the anatomist Thomas Willis, a contemporary of Christopher Wren, attempted to explain hysteria in similar terms.[23,24]

The spiritual father of neuropsychiatry, Wilhelm Greisinger, set the modern agenda for the field in Germany during the nineteenth century. His 1845 monograph, *Mental Pathology and Therapeutics*, made the central tenet of neuropsychiatry explicit. By asserting that psychiatric disorders are really brain diseases,[25] Greisinger put forth a clear hypothesis that no one could misconstrue. His ideas guided many like-minded psychiatrists who followed him. They pursued neuropsychiatry in search of evidence to support his claims. The British physician Henry Maudsley, for instance, elaborated Greisinger's views in 1867 by pointing out the dependence of brain activity on chemical substrates and proposed that mental illness might reflect chemical abnormalities.

In 1913, Hideyo Noguchi, a Japanese bacteriologist working in America,[26] greatly boosted the prestige of neuropsychiatry by demonstrating for the first time that at least one physical agent in the brain could produce psychological illness. Neurological symptoms like headache and muscle weakness had been connected with the venereal disease called syphilis since medieval times. Reports of a variant exhibiting mental symptoms had appeared in the medical literature at the end of the eighteenth century. Possible causes of neurosyphilis thereafter began to assume importance because of its psychiatric reputation as the "great imitator"; the malady was associated with a panoply of problems including amnesia, violence, depression, mania, delusions, and paranoia.[27–29]

Investigators like Bayle in the 1820s had identified abnormalities within the nervous systems of victims who died of syphilis. Three quarters of a century later, physicians were able to use fluid drained from the spinal column to reveal evidence of inflamed membranes around the brains of live patients with the disease. Alois Alzheimer in 1904 characterized the germane brain cell changes caused by syphilis. In 1906, August von Wassermann developed a diagnostic blood test for the illness. Noguchi's work in 1913 actually showed *Treponema*, the microorganism known to produce syphilis, in the brains of affected individuals, including those with mental symptoms. During World War I, Wagner-Jauregg originated the induction of fever as a therapy for the illness. World War II introduced penicillin as a definitive cure not only for neurosyphilis but also for many other infectious processes.[30-36]

Joseph Goldberger pioneered another line of research lending clout to neuropsychiatry. In 1914, he traced the cause of pellagra, which produces behavioral disturbances, to diet after noting that institutional patients but not staff suffered from the disease. Goldberger altered the contents of meals in ways that reproduced and then eliminated pellagra, thereby identifying particular food components as critical in the development and treatment of the disease. His animal research produced the theory, verified by later workers, that amino acid and vitamin deficiencies cause the pellagra syndrome.[37]

Emil Kraepelin and his neuropsychiatric coterie were flourishing at this time. Kraepelin had made his reputation among German psychiatrists at the end of the nineteenth century and the beginning of the twentieth. After an education in Würzburg, he had become a professor at several different universities. A stint with the innovative psychologist Wilhelm Wundt had given him a marked experimental bias. When Kraepelin finally was appointed psychiatric director at the medical school in Munich, his department filled up with brain researchers. Alzheimer, who investigated not only syphilis but also the dementing illness now named after him, worked in Munich. So did Nissl, who invented a method of coloring nerve tissue to make it visible under the microscope, and Brodmann, who mapped varying nerve cell patterns in different parts of the brain. Neuroscientists came to dominate other German-speaking faculties as well, including Sigmund Freud's alma mater in Vienna. By the time Kraepelin died in 1926, the commitment of academic German psychiatrists lay squarely in the neurological camp.[38-41]

Practicing physicians did not necessarily share the neuropsychiatric outlook common in medical schools. Freud left the academic fold, opened a private office, and finally abandoned all attempts to link his own brand of psychotherapy to the brain. His famous theories gave rise to many mentalistic schools of psychology[42-44] that completely ignored the brain and found wide popular appeal.

Behind the scenes, however, academicians lay waiting for a series of discoveries that would catapult brain advocates into the driver's seat. New biological treatments for mental illness with direct effects on brain function filled the bill.[45] A growing number of people began to ferret out strictly medical therapies that promised to outdo the "talking cures" of Freud and company.[46]

The first modern methods proved to be crude, useless, or dangerous. In 1929, neuroses were treated unsuccessfully with carbon dioxide gas. Four years later, Manfred Sakel used insulin injections to produce temporary coma, which he thought might help schizophrenic patients. Many experimental subjects awakened with permanent brain damage, so the technique was abandoned.[47]

At about that time, workers at Yale University showed that certain types of brain surgery calmed experimental chimpanzees. A Portuguese investigator named Egas Moniz exploited this information in 1935 by performing frontal lobotomies on 20 psychotic people. Their mental symptoms improved after surgery, leading American medical centers to adopt the technique for use on their own human patients. Inventive surgeons soon simplified the procedure to "cingulotomy," a less disruptive operation that replaced the more extensive lobotomy for selected psychiatric conditions. Moniz won a Nobel Prize for his original work.[48,49]

The permanent impact of brain operations on behavior, however, soon led to a demand for more reversible therapies. The first of these therapies was prompted by anecdotal accounts of improvement in schizophrenic symptoms after accidents that had produced convulsive seizures. In 1934, a Hungarian named Lazlo Von Meduna, inspired by such reports, purposely used injections of camphor and later pentylenetetrazol to cause brief convulsions as a treatment for psychiatric patients. Several years later, Ugo Cerletti and Lucio Bini in Italy found a way to bring on fits without the need for injections. They applied an electric current to the scalp and stimulated seizures. The result was relief of some mental symptoms, particularly in depressed subjects.

Efforts were made to reduce disturbing side effects, but, not surprisingly, to its opponents electroshock still seemed as ghoulish a technique as lobotomy.[50] In response, drug treatments that sidestepped any need for convulsions sprang up after World War II.

An Australian researcher named John Cade found that salts of the element lithium pacified laboratory guinea pigs. This prompted him in 1949 to study the effect of lithium on humans in frenzied states; his measures controlled the agitation of some patients. During the next two decades, other investigators, including Mogens Schau in Denmark, repeated Cade's work with particular success in treating acute manic excitement. Consequently, oral administration of lithium spread throughout Europe, Great Britain, and, by 1970, the United States.[51,52]

Three years after the Australian lithium trial, French researchers came up with their own claims to fame. Henri Laborit had experimented with a substance called promethazine as a supplement to surgical anaesthesia, hoping that it would prevent circulatory collapse.[53] He failed in his original aim, but in the process he noticed that the drug had quieting influences on behavior. Furthermore, unlike sedatives previously known to doctors, promethazine seemed to tranquilize patients without making them fall asleep. Laborit later tested a derivative compound, chlorpromazine, which produced similar but more pronounced effects.

These observations inspired Jean Delay and Paul Deniker in 1952 to try chlorpromazine as a treatment for severely disturbed psychiatric patients. The drug appeared to reduce agitated behavior, delusions, and hallucinations in a variety of mental illnesses, including mania, depression, and schizophrenia. Subsequently, others repeated the work and went on to develop over 20 related compounds. These became a mainstay of therapy for the acute phases of many psychotic disorders.[54,55]

An experimental substance originally slated for use against

tuberculosis became the first antidepressant through a similar series of events. A medical worker testing iproniazid happened to notice that it made patients euphoric. Though further experience linked the drug to dangerous side effects, the positive actions of iproniazid prompted a search for safer mood-improving agents. One innovative pharmaceutical company had meanwhile fashioned chlorpromazine into a new chemical, imipramine, which it was hoped would surpass its parent as a tranquilizer. In 1958, Roland Kuhn more accurately identified imipramine as a potential antidepressant. It turned out not to have many of iproniazid's flaws. Kuhn's observations cleared the way for drug firms to develop other medications active against depression. These include such drugs as amitriptyline, desipramine, doxepine, trazodone, and fluoxetine.[56–58]

Even minor neuroses, which Freud had tried to cure with his talking therapies, evolved into a target for pills and elixirs. Bromides, chloral hydrate, barbiturates, meprobamates, and benzodiazepines have all taken their turns in the treatment of anxiety. For some special neurotic conditions, other substances like clomipramine have recently come into vogue.[59,60]

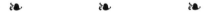

More than any other factor, these developments now feed the hope that neurological research will do away with mental illness. The role of agents like chlorpromazine in liberating chronic patients from psychiatric hospitals[61] has fired a hunger to understand how existing drugs work and might be perfected. Psychiatrists once happy to leave less curable diagnoses in the murky arena of mind now feel a duty to move them toward the brain, where chemistry and electrical probing seem to promise miraculous solutions.

Neuropsychiatric advocates expect that not only mental disability but also its shame will disappear through its redefinition as a physical disease. They cite the once trendy concept of "schizophrenogenesis" as a source of unnecessary stigma for families of psychotic patients. It assigned "painful culpability" to the conduct of parents who, before modern neuropsychiatry, were blamed for driving their schizophrenic children crazy. Newer evidence for biological causes of the disease, however, has ostensibly relieved at least some of this parental guilt. Neuropsychiatric "reconceptualization" thus reveals itself as a putative source of humanism in the care of mental disease.[62,63]

Hence, even in America, old German academic traditions are finally sweeping into control. The schism that Dr. Kandel described is thus closing, with the balance tilted in favor of neuropsychiatrists. Today, the inheritors of Wilhelm Greisinger's nineteenth-century viewpoint, right or wrong, are clearly in global ascendency.[64] A recent Act of Congress dubbing the 1990s "the Decade of the Brain" symbolizes the trend.

A mass of facts speaks for itself. New scholarly neuropsychiatric societies have recently banded together under the auspices of academicians from leading American medical schools. Many such organizations produce neuropsychiatric publications, which have proliferated over recent decades. Among psychiatric journals on the shelves of a major medical school library, the author found that the average neurologically oriented periodical is ten years younger than those with more traditional kinds of subject matter. Several new publications explicitly using the word "neuropsychiatry" in their titles have appeared within the last ten years. These include exhaustive new textbooks and journals that feature contributions by elite researchers.

Even general psychiatric literature has become more oriented toward the brain. One premier journal published 126 articles during the first half of 1988; 24 percent of them dealt with neuroscientific issues. In comparison, only 9 percent directly concerned the brain 10 years earlier.

There is evidence that not only public practices and politics, but also the privately held theories of psychiatrists today are becoming more like those of Greisinger. A recent survey of physicians in a major psychiatric teaching institution revealed that residents were 27 percent more likely than older psychiatrists to embrace neuropsychiatric biases about the nature of mental processes and disorders. Another survey conducted at a comparable medical center also suggested that youth and recent training correlate with biological biases in psychiatric practice habits.

Many brain science advocates feel bold enough to expand these trends into a training revolution that will make the grip of neurobiology on American psychiatry unbreakable. At least one spokesperson has advocated abandoning the study of mind in psychiatry altogether in favor of an exclusive educational focus on the brain. He has decried the idea of a psychiatrist with no training in anatomy or physiology beyond medical school. He has strongly argued for the formulation of a new kind of psychiatric residency with apprenticeships in medicine, neurology, drug chemistry, neuropsychology, electrophysiology, and radiological techniques for imaging the brain. He has set as a goal for such training the creation of a future psychiatric cadre whose members identify themselves as neuroscientists. He has advised that old, outmoded, shaman-like skills of psychiatry, not connected to any knowledge of the brain, be relegated to a course for medical students on interviewing techniques and legal matters. He has suggested that only through such changes will future psychiatrists be equipped to create viable, neurobiological theories of mental illness.

Neuropsychiatrists, justifying these kinds of views with the vaunted efficiency of their methods, expect that through the impact of biological therapy, humanity will finally abolish mental disorders. At first glance, this vision seems appealing. Neat readouts from gleaming new laboratories will unlock the secrets of human nature. Madness, with all the pain, poverty, deluded thinking, family disarray, and self-abuse that it implies, will melt away before the clarity of brain science. The messy verbal groping and mental masturbation of Freudian therapy, which can drag on for years and makes no promises for a cure, will end. One might expect few people of conscience to reject this kind of utopia.

It is no wonder, then, that the modern promise of neuropsychiatry has already begun to attract a large army of true believers, many of them powerful and articulate. As we have seen, the movement has defined its canons, carved out an expanding beach-head, and encircled its opponents. But like any juggernaut, its gathering momentum threatens to escape control, and its less realistic assumptions may do unforeseen damage. The time is right for a closer look at the underpinnings of neuropsychiatric thinking, in order to detect any hidden flaws.

2

Neuropsychiatry's Current State

*I*n recent years, an avalanche of data, comprising more than 95 percent of all the brain findings ever linked to behavior, has inundated psychiatry.[1] New investigative tools have uncovered a vast storehouse of measurable brain oddities that correlate seductively with classical psychiatric syndromes. In particular, state-of-the-art computerized scanners[2-4] now provide increasingly fine resolution of brain images that have led to a bonanza of apparent empirical support for the neuropsychiatric school of thought.

The prototypical modern brain scanning systems, called computerized tomography (CT) machines, employ X-ray photography coupled to software algorithms that have vastly improved the kinds of pictures available to radiologists. An Austrian, J. Radon, who was trying to solve problems related to gravitational fields in outer space, first created the mathematical basis of CT technology as a by-product of his research in 1917. Research in solar astronomy and electron microscopy during later decades produced refinements of Radon's concepts. Between 1956 and 1963, a South African researcher named A. M. Cormack used related ideas to show that computers could be harnessed to radiation detectors arrayed at multiple sites around the outside of the human body in order to extract internal anatomical data. G. N. Hounsfield, an engineer at English Musical Instruments, Ltd., in Great Britain, then made the critical leap in designing a practical CT device.

W. H. Oldendorf built a prototype machine in 1961; Hounsfield and Comack shared the 1979 Nobel Prize for their work. Scanning in a clinical setting first began at Atkinson Morley's Hospital in Wimbledon in 1971. The first published data concerning patients appeared in 1973, when commercial scanners went into general use. Progressive upgrades in machine design followed.[5]

Even sharper likenesses of the brain became available in the 1980s through the magnetic resonance imager (MRI), which harnesses electromagnetic waves to examine brain structure in live human subjects. Bloch and Purcell had discovered the principle of resonance for atoms placed in a magnetic field in 1946. They received the 1952 Nobel Prize for their efforts, which found application in laboratory chemical analysis during the 1950s and 1960s. In the 1970s, Damadian, Lauterbur, and others pioneered the marriage of CT-like computer algorithms to nuclear magnetic resonance and hence produced diagnostic imaging machines capable of astonishing clarity.[6,7]

A different generation of scanners called positron and single-photon emission tomography (PET and SPECT) machines were developed to assess function rather than simple structure in particular brain regions. The idea of SPECT and PET imaging wedded the computer algorithms of CT scanning to radioisotope tracing techniques that follow brain physiology as outlined by Kety and Schmidt in 1948 and Lassen and Monk in 1955. Kuhl and Edwards used these principles in constructing a crude forerunner of SPECT and PET machines in 1963. In the late 1970s and 1980s, progress in this kind of approach accelerated rapidly.[8,9] Modern SPECT and PET devices are now able to pinpoint the rate at which radioactively labeled blood flows through each part of the brain. Their readouts can also analyze the speed at which different brain structures consume calories in sugar molecules attached to radioisotopes.

Still newer instruments, "fast" MRI machines, promise to outdo even SPECT and PET scanning. SPECT and PET images are somewhat blurred; they also require injection of radioactive drugs whose cumulative side effects limit the repeatability of studies on the same subject. The new "fast" MRI scanners may bypass these difficulties in the near future.[10–12]

CT images, MRI scans, and correlated autopsy findings all appear to link mental symptoms with abnormal brain anatomy. Among a subgroup of severely schizophrenic subjects, for example, scans have shown that the entire brain shrinks. Patients with this finding tend to have more deadpan emotional styles and poorer responses to drugs than those with normal scans. Scientists have reported particularly shriveled tissue in the hindbrain of some schizophrenics.[13–15] PET and SPECT machines have also detected signs of impaired circulation and sugar metabolism in frontal regions of schizophrenic brains. Abnormal patterns have appeared in patients with mood disorders, panic attacks, and Alzheimer's disease as well.[16–26] Researchers plan to exploit fast MRI technology in order to solidify such functional imaging data and study other aspects of psychiatric disease.[27–29]

ða   ða   ða

The relationship of mental illness to the brain's chemical balance has been spotlighted by many contemporary laboratory techniques even without imaging. For example, neuroscientists have been able to link the substance dopamine to abnormalities in schizophrenic frontal lobes. They note that autopsies have turned up an excess of dopamine "receptors" in relevant regions of schizophrenic brains and that persons with physical diseases affecting dopamine sites may show schizophrenic behaviors. It has been learned that drugs like amphetamine, which boost the influence of dopamine on the brain, worsen schizophrenic symptoms, while other agents like chlorpromazine, which prevent dopamine from reaching its receptor sites, may improve the clinical picture. Schizophrenic patients also harbor large amounts of another chemical called norepinephrine in parts of their forebrains, and drugs that affect norepinephrine may influence schizophrenic symptoms.[30–33]

Norepinephrine has suspected links to a second illness, depression, and breaks down into the chemical 3-methoxy-4-hydroxy-phenylglycol (MHPG) before leaving the body through the kidneys. Scientists have noted low MHPG levels in the urine of some depressed subjects; they have therefore concluded that brain norepinephrine during depression is also low. Reductions in another substance, 5-hydroxyindole acetic acid (5-HIAA), originating from the breakdown of the brain chemical serotonin, have been seen in the spinal fluid of depressed patients. A number of researchers have found that drugs known to affect both norepinephrine and serotonin aggravate mania and relieve depression. Scientists thus perceive a tantalizing connection between the two chemicals, with deficits of both norepinephrine and serotonin evident in some depressed patients.[34,35]

Researchers have furnished further data on brain chemistry's link with depression. Chemical assays have revealed high amounts of a compound called cortisol in the blood of depressed persons. A maneuver known as the dexamethasone suppression test (DST) suggests that these cortisol excesses involve the brain. Additional probes of brain chemistry, including the so-called insulin tolerance test and thyrotropin-releasing hormone (TRH) stimulation test, follow the same pattern.[36]

Brain chemicals linked to pathological violence include serotonin, norepinephrine, dopamine, acetyl choline, gamma-aminobutyric acid (GABA), testosterone, and the opioids.[37] In particular, scientists have come up with evidence that ties aggressive and self-abusive conduct to reduced serotonin levels[38]: Violent patients appear to have shortages of the serotonin by-product 5-HIAA, and drugs that increase serotonin activity sometimes reduce aggressive and suicidal acts. Impulsive behavior, particularly violence, also occurs with increased norepinephrine activity: Surpluses of norepinephrine by-products appear in some impulsive patients, stimulants augmenting norepinephrine's actions increase aggressive conduct, and drugs blocking norepinephrine effects inhibit assaultive behavior.

Links between mental symptoms and additional sorts of biological parameters have emerged. Correlations have been found between schizophrenia, viral antibodies, and seasonally relevant epidemiological data.[39,40] "EEG" machines have provided evidence of electrical changes in the brain activity of selected mental patients.[41,42] In the field of genetics, increased risks for mood disorders, schizophrenia, and antisocial behavior have surfaced among twins and other relatives of mental patients. An especially well-known series of research studies found an abnormal amount of psychiatric illness in children of disturbed mothers after they had been separated at birth by adoption. Even normal behavioral traits have been tied to genetic factors.[43–46]

Neurologists have discovered that a broad spectrum of abnormal brain processes traditionally classified as strictly physical illnesses can in fact produce conduct mimicking psychiatric conditions. Patients with multiple sclerosis often seem to show extreme shifts in mood, poor contact with reality, and socially inappropriate humor. Blows to the head appear to make people irritable, resulting in a pattern called the posttraumatic syndrome. Fifty percent of all brain tumor cases show signs of a psychiatric disturbance. Birth trauma, malnutrition, head injuries, and constitutional sensitivity to alcohol all correlate with pathologically violent behavior. Parkinson's disease, epileptic seizures, and many other neurological problems have proved to be associated with mood changes, disordered thoughts, and other mental symptoms.[47–52]

Neurologists have related specific psychiatric symptoms to physical damage in distinct places within the brain. Observers have noted, for example, that injury to the left frontal brain surface often produces depression, while pathology deep within the right side of the brain can lead to mania. Impulsive and pseudo-schizophrenic behavior has been found to accompany some forms of injury to the brain's frontal and temporal regions. Violence correlates with damage to the frontal and so-called "limbic"[53] brain structures.[54–59]

Researchers have found that totally extraneural medical illnesses can affect the brain and hence mimic psychiatric conditions. Examples include hormone storms, palpitations, low blood sugar, pneumonia, menstrual irregularities, vitamin B_{12} deficiency, cancer of the pancreas, faulty excretion of copper, and deranged immune function.[60,61]

Ongoing refinements in drug therapy for psychiatric symptoms[62,63] have encouraged the neuropsychiatric viewpoint. A recent journal article suggests that we are now so advanced in the art of psychopharmacology that present research challenges pertain mainly to mere "fine tuning" of existing chemotherapeutic agents.[64]

As a result of all these developments, today's psychiatrists find neurological biases nearly irresistible. Evidence from such sources as neuroanatomical dissections, biochemical tests, computerized scans, neuropsychological examinations, and pharmacotherapeutics[65] inspires theoretical models of psychiatric disease focused on neuroanatomy, transmitter chemistry, electrical brain disturbances, genetics, and even viruses.[66]

For example, one group of researchers has explained schizophrenia by advancing the so-called dopamine theory, which claims that schizophrenia is caused by the increased chemical activity of dopamine.[67] Another theory about schizophrenia suggests excessive norepinephrine as the causal agent. A third theory places the blame for schizophrenia not on particular substances but instead on frontal lobe dysfunction. A fourth points its finger at schizophrenogenic brain scars that form during birth trauma.

Psychiatric experts have also attributed mania and depression to chemical abnormalities in the brain. Many implicate norepinephrine, others serotonin. Still other investigators have theorized that mania may arise in a manner similar to epilepsy, feeding on itself with each repeated attack of symptoms.

Current neuropsychiatric opinion links even neurotic anxiety to the disturbed brain chemistry of substances like norepinephrine, serotonin, and GABA.[68–72] But the most innovatively biological view of all proposes that biological defects cause not only the acute symptoms of schizophrenia, manic–depressive illness, aggressive behavioral syndromes, and neuroses; the same biological causes ostensibly operate on a continuum that also extends into the chronic realm of personality disturbances, traditionally viewed as non-biological.[73,74] This theory asserts that serotonin deficits and norepinephrine overactivity underlie habitually impulsive behavior, that oversensitivity to norepinephrine or acetylcholine causes ongoing mood instability, and that abnormalities in norepinephrine or GABA contribute to chronic anxiety.[75]

       ꙳   ꙳   ꙳

The main body of empirical data in neuropsychiatry has been obtained through good and conscientious work. Nonetheless, it also appears to harbor flaws. These flaws stem not only from practical limits on the data-gathering power of existing scanners, chemical tests, and other laboratory equipment. Basic theoretical paradigms are at fault as well. Resulting findings and conclusions therefore contain holes.

For instance, no single biological hypothesis regarding the causes of schizophrenia explains all relevant empirical data. No one theory has yet reconciled evidence that supports alternative dopamine and norepinephrine hypotheses. Furthermore, the role of dopamine by itself is a messy issue. The substance is present in several different regions of the brain. Drugs like chlorpromazine, which in the laboratory block the impact of dopamine on neurons quite rapidly, act much more sluggishly on symptoms at the clinical level. Furthermore, chlorpromazine's effects extend in a confusing way beyond schizophrenia to other psychiatric illnesses. These facts complicate any simple link between dopamine and schizophrenia.[76–79]

Anatomical theories about schizophrenia falter when limited empirical data are invoked to sort through a complex morass of causes and effects. Several brain sites may be involved in a particular functional derangement; it is not always clear which locus directs the others. Moreover, abnormal findings in the brains of psychiatric patients cannot suffice to show that underlying anatomical lesions have created mental disorders. Investigators must also consider the matter in reverse—the possibility that mental illnesses such as schizophrenia, perhaps through poor nutritional habits, themselves sometimes produce brain lesions or even chemical abnormalities.[80]

Evidence for the role of genes in schizophrenia remains incomplete. The coincidence of schizophrenia in identical twins is high but not 100 percent. Experts have suggested both "environmental factors" and incomplete gene expression to fill this statistical gap.[81] Such explanations at present cannot be proven or refuted by experiment. One gene may influence many traits, and many genes may converge on one trait.[82] Some "genes" don't even operate as genes: Less than 5 percent of DNA encodes specific proteins, and the function of the remainder is not entirely clear.[83] No one today can sort through all possible pathways to broken neurons from "sick" DNA.[84]

Serious flaws undermine theories not only about schizophrenia but also about mood disorders. Though many would like to identify a lack of norepinephrine or serotonin in the brain as the cause of depression, some drugs able to boost the impact of these substances treat depressive symptoms poorly. Other agents that work well as antidepressants have doubtful effects on brain chemicals like norepinephrine and serotonin. Particularly troublesome for chemical explanations of mood disorders is the realization that abnormal DST results, once considered a hallmark of depression, are in fact neither sensitive nor specific as a sign of the illness; "diagnostic" findings do not appear in all depressed patients and may occur during healthy, nondepressed grief reactions.[85-87]

No one has proved that any biological factor corresponds exactly to tendencies toward pathological violence. Although some people who commit violent crimes also demonstrate evidence of brain dysfunction, many exhibit no such abnormalities. Furthermore, most people with brain diseases do not act violently. It is often difficult when studying aggressive subjects via neuropsychological tests to untangle the relative contributions of brain damage, antisocial personality disorders, depression, and boredom. Over the long haul, gender has not correlated well with assaultive behavior in psychiatric patients. It has proved impossible to isolate neuroelectrical disturbances as a critical factor in purposive criminal violence. Searches in the brain for a particular site that regulates violence and for one chemical responsible for all aggression have failed. Overall, no single specific factor[88] accurately predicts violent behavior in the long run, and neither drugs nor surgical interventions have provided truly reliable remedies. The normal statistical curve along which tendencies toward violence vary in human beings remains only a description defying neuroscientific explanation or cure.[89–92]

る。   る。   る。

The great psychiatrist Adolph Meyer (1866–1950) opposed "narrowing mind-shy" influences of mechanistic thinking in his field. He particularly abhorred the limited perspective of strictly biological theories.[93] Although he was educated as a laboratory neuropathologist in Switzerland, Meyer moved beyond such materialistic horizons after he emigrated in 1892. In the United States, at Kankakee State Hospital, he became interested in clinical psychiatric phenomena and the personal difficulties of patients. Immersion in the philosophies of such American thinkers as John Dewey and Charles Sanders Peirce led Meyer to reject schemes that sort the psychic afflictions of people into rigid categories of mental "diseases" analogous to somatic disorders. Instead, Meyer tried to look closely at the overall life history of each individual patient. This approach produced therapeutic successes that propelled Meyer into directorial posts at Worcester Hospital, the New York State Psychiatric Institute, and finally Johns Hopkins University. He became a leading voice in American psychiatry through the 1940s.[94]

Meyer would be among the first to tell us today that although neuropsychiatric concepts may sometimes help in understanding the mind, they are hardly ever sufficient.[95] He might suggest that our very tendency to see normal and abnormal human consciousness solely in terms of material processes creates the flaws that compromise current neuropsychiatric research.

He might also remind us that nonbiological psychotherapy

is, in its own way, very effective. A study by the National Institutes of Health has demonstrated the usefulness of interpersonal psychotherapy in depression.[96] Insight-oriented psychotherapy remains the first-line treatment for several personality disorders and neuroses.[97,98] A form of psychotherapy even has its place in psychosis.[99] Research by the Civilian Health and Medical Program of the Uniformed Services, data from the Blue Cross Federal Employees Plan, and a meta-analysis of 58 other surveys have shown that outpatient psychotherapy saves money by reducing the frequency of psychiatric hospitalizations and medical illnesses.[100]

It is important to keep these facts in mind, because potential ethical fallout from today's eclipse of the psyche by neuroscience has serious negative implications.[101] Neuropsychiatric monomania can impel clinicians to treat patients summarily as diagnostic categories instead of individual people. It encourages what Philadelphia psychoanalyst Elio Frattaroli calls "the quick fix" that "threatens not only psychotherapy but rational pharmacotherapy as well."[102-104] Washington neurologist Richard Restak points out that the grandiose project of painting all abnormal behavior as brain disease can "threaten to eliminate the . . . concept of . . . a rational being endowed with . . . responsibilities."[105] Among other dangers, there lurks the possibility of thereby turning a patient's individuality into an impersonal bag of molecules.

Thomas Szasz, a University of Chicago–trained professor of psychiatry at the State University of New York in Syracuse and author of over 100 books,[106] has expressed these sorts of concerns most cogently. He writes that

the notion of a person "having a mental illness" . . . provides professional assent to a popular rationalization—namely that problems in living experienced and expressed in terms of so-called psychiatric symptoms are basically similar to bodily diseases. Moreover, the concept . . . undermines the principle of personal responsibility. . . . For the individual, the notion of mental illness precludes an inquiring attitude toward his conflict which his "symptoms" at once conceal and reveal. For a society, it precludes regarding individuals as responsible persons and invites, instead, treating them as irresponsible patients.[107]

Neuropsychiatric methods, particularly those based on medication, foster an atmosphere in which the doctor takes control instead of helping the patient control himself as much as possible.[108–110] Surrender of personal autonomy by patients can have profoundly negative consequences. Since physicians are only human, and since any one of us runs the risk of falling ill, giving doctors too much control over patients opens all of us to errors in treatment. Such mistakes may involve physical manipulations undertaken in the ostensible interests of patients.[111]

Pharmacotherapy[112] is a particularly pointed lesson in this regard. Drugs are variably effective in all areas of medicine, but doctors often overprescribe them. Every drug carries some risk of toxic side effects. While advances in chemical treatments specifically for mental illness have lent credence to the neuropsychiatric viewpoint, they also create their own especially serious problems. No one knows whether any of the new psychiatric drugs when chronically ingested will cause long-term, cumulative side effects; it is simply too soon to tell.[113] Addiction is a particular hazard of many psychoactive substances already in general use.[114]

Addictive sedatives are an easy way for a doctor to control his patients' anxieties. As short-term remedies, they work faster and more predictably than mere "talk therapy." However, a long-term chemical dependency can often enslave patients more completely than do their illnesses.

Abuse of chemical agents, including psychiatric prescription drugs, has become epidemic in the United States. Some clinicians never seem to learn that materialistic balms for emotional pain not only fail to solve psychological problems, but also may rebound to multiply them,[115] even to the extent of reducing autonomous patients to addicts. Research to curb abuse potential through

biochemical modifications most often backfires: Different generations of sedatives, including barbiturates, carbamates, piperidine-
diones, and benzodiazepines, have all proven addictive after sustained use. Nonetheless, each new generation of addictive drugs
has found its way into the arsenal of pills that too many doctors
give their anxious patients for a "quick fix."

Strictly neurobiological approaches to mental illness, in creating such serious traps, kill human freedom in the process. This
happens because, like all technical instruments, neurobiological
tools tempt the people who use them with a physical ability to
control others.[116] Anyone, whether medically trained or not, may
cave in to the appeal of such absolute power. For this reason,
neuropsychiatry can augment the tendency of all technology to
extend its dry methods from laboratory surrogates into the very
soul of man.[117]

Hence, although modern neuropsychiatry has both good and
bad aspects, ill effects are growing with particular rapidity. It is
certainly true that neuroscience has come up with powerful drugs
to limit or reduce many psychiatric symptoms. Neuropsychiatrists have also used new imaging and biochemical technology to
learn a host of facts about brain–behavior correlations in health
and disease. On the negative side, however, some biologically
oriented enthusiasts have gone overboard in claiming that brain
processes are the exclusive causes of mental pathology. These
claims ignore major gaps in the evidence, especially those that
blur boundaries between cause and effect. Neuropsychiatric ex-
tremism has led to overuse of drugs and other expedients that
endanger patient autonomy. Such problems are on the rise as
neuroscience edges toward a monopolistic hold on the minds of
psychiatrists.

3

Neuropsychiatry and the Philosophy of Mind

*W*e have seen that neuropsychiatry produces problematic empirical data, research designs, clinical practices, and, most importantly, ethical implications. However, its negative philosophical impact is more than ethical; neuropsychiatry distorts other aspects of philosophy as well.

The discipline of philosophy is divided into "value-laden" and "value-free" branches. The value-laden portions consist of ethics, aesthetics, and political philosophy, while value-free parts include logic, epistemology, and ontology. Ethics addresses questions of moral value, aesthetics probes the artistic value of beauty, and political philosophy investigates social values. Logic plumbs the laws of rational inference, epistemology asks how knowledge is possible, and ontology studies the nature of existence.[1]

We cannot ignore the flawed ontology flowing from neuropsychiatric biases.[2] It is to this issue that we now turn.

The most simple-minded ontological assumption used to justify the neuropsychiatric viewpoint is the doctrine that a material foundation underlies all mental states. Anyone embracing this idea must try to understand the human mind by tracing its building blocks to more and more fundamental physical components. At a university, he or she might construct a relevant program of study by starting with psychology but moving in logical, orderly succession into biology, chemistry, and finally physics. Such a program would shift the student's objects of scrutiny from thoughts to behavior, behavior to physiology, physiology to biochemistry, and biochemistry to the physics of relevant atoms. Hence, the material origins of the mind might be expected to reveal themselves.

The doctrine that a material foundation underlies all mental states has a long history. Several ancient Greek thinkers furnished its basis by describing all reality as some form of matter. Thales chose water as his bedrock for reality. Anaximenes picked air, and Empedocles lumped both water and air together with solid earthen matter.[3] Leucippus (450–420 BC) described all reality as moving particulate matter in the first "atomic" account of nature. His junior colleague, Democritus of Abdera (460–370 BC), the so-called "Laughing Philosopher," enunciated these ideas loudly enough to make them last millenia: Democritus' claims were the main topic of Karl Marx's Ph.D. dissertation more than 2000 years later.[4–7]

In Roman times, Galen augmented Greek materialism with his own idea that a material vapor or liquid animates the body.[8] During the sixteenth century, an alchemist called Paracelsus (1493–1541) advanced an allied view that all life processes are chemical in nature.[9] Paracelsus was the pseudonym of Theophrastus Bombastus von Hohenheim, an intellectual adventurer born to the family of a physician in Einsiedeln, Switzerland. He attended Basel University, learned the art of alchemy from the Bishop of Würzburg, and thereafter traveled about Europe picking up a wealth of local information about medical practice. Paracelsus's burgeoning healing skills brought him fame; he was appointed town physician and university medical lecturer in Basel. However, his innovative ideas about chemotherapeutics contradicted the prevailing orthodoxies of his day. He was therefore expelled from Basel in 1528 and again became a wanderer.[10]

A century later, Thomas Hobbes (1588–1679) refined the views of Paracelsus and others by reducing not just simple life processes but actual complex thoughts to discrete motions of minute particles.[11–14] The strict rigor of Hobbes's ideas reflected a mind trained at Oxford from the age of 15. At 22, he encountered the writings of Johannes Kepler, whose physics began converting him to a materialistic viewpoint. He also began serving as tutor to a nobleman, William Cavendish, who introduced him to such scientific luminaries as Francis Bacon. After Cavendish's death, Hobbes traveled to Paris and to Italy, where he personally met the physicist Galileo Galilei and cemented his own materialism. In 1651, Hobbes published his best-known work, the *Leviathan*, whose content ran afoul of the French monarchy and led the English governments of Cromwell and the Restoration to silence him.[15,16]

The views of two French Enlightenment thinkers, Julien Offray de la Mettrie (1709–1751) and Baron Paul Heinrich Dietrich d'Holbach (1723–1789), picked up on Hobbes's ideas by reducing the universe and man as part of it to moving physical objects.[17] The seventeenth-century English neuroanatomist Thomas Willis assumed this same perspective in his concept of a "spiritous humour" consisting of particles migrating through nerves. A later Swiss professor of anatomy and physiology in Göttingen, Albrecht Von Haller (1708–1777), voiced similar beliefs; he suggested that sensation and volition derive from a "liquor" flowing between the brain and the body's periphery.[18,19]

In our century, modern inheritors of Leucippus, Democritus, Galen, Hobbes, de la Mettrie, d'Holbach, Willis, and Von Haller have spun many variations from the materialist paradigm. For example, the Australian philosophers J. J. C. Smart and David Armstrong have espoused a theory positing that mental and neural domains of reality are identical.[20,21] Their colleague, U. T. Place, has claimed that the idea of consciousness as a material brain process is a scientifically testable hypothesis contingent on empirical facts, just as one can verify by experiment that a cloud consists of water droplets.[22–24] "Epiphenomenalist" philosophers[25] have asserted that mind constitutes only a mirage arising as an accidental by-product of material processes; psychosomatic traffic thus appears to flow only in a single causal direction, from body to mind.[26–29]

"Eliminativistic" materialists have pushed the outright idea that mentality, mirage or not, simply does not exist. Exponents like Richard Rorty have gone as far as suggesting that when both mental and neural terms exist for the same phenomenon, scientific precision requires that neural terms completely supplant mental ones.[30] The goal of eliminativism is to purge psychology of all but its own materialistic explanations for behavior.[31,32]

           ɜ▲   ɜ▲   ɜ▲

Materialists, particularly in more recent times, have justified their philosophical position by citing all the empirical successes of neuroscience in accounting for human behavior. We have seen, however, that these successes are flawed. Yet even if all the empirical data now known by brain science could support the contentions of biological psychiatry, its summed weight would never guarantee total triumph of neuropsychiatric models in the unknown future. Correlating specific mental and neural events in the present can never seal their connection for all time.[33] As Sir John Eccles has explained, faith that the psychobiological approach will ultimately explain the entire domain of mind is

> simply a religious belief held by dogmatic materialists who often confuse their religion with their science. It has all the feature of a messianic prophesy with the promise of a future free from all problems—a kind of nirvana for our unfortunate successors.[34]

Such "promissory" defects in support for materialism relate to its basis in circular reasoning. Neuroscientific research backs up philosophical materialism, but materialism justifies that research in the first place. This circularity undercuts the entire future of the neuropsychiatric paradigm.

Materialism is beset by other flaws as well. Since it provides for no causal influence of mind on matter, materialism gives us no way to understand how mind has helped man survive the material processes of natural selection. The definition of matter itself turns out to be a difficult task, as Einstein's equivalence of mass and energy illustrates.[35,36]

Of course, there has always been opposition to materialistic excesses among philosophers. The philosophical school of idealism has offered a variety of rebuttals and alternatives. Among the ancient Greeks, for instance, Anaximander pointed to an elusive entity called the "unlimited" as sole organizing principle of the universe. Plato sought a foundation in his concept of the "Good,"[37] and Anaxagoras conceived of mind itself as the basis of reality.

A much later idealist, Bishop George Berkeley, tried to retain a vestigial notion of matter, yet undercut its solidity by explaining the objective world as a kind of "concept" in the mind of God. This perspective reflected the sort of tensions that suffused Berkeley's entire life. He was born in 1685 in Kilkenny, Ireland, but his parents were of English lineage. Berkeley attended Kilkenny College and Trinity College in Dublin, where he was exposed to the cutting edge in philosophical thought of his day, and visited the cosmopolitan city of London. Yet he also remained connected to his church throughout his life. He was appointed Dean of Derry in 1724. After a three-year trip to Rhode Island to promote a project attempting to establish a missionary college in Burmuda, Berkeley returned to Ireland and was made Bishop of Cloyne in 1734. He made substantial efforts on behalf of his poorer parishioners until his retirement to Oxford in 1752 and death the following year.

Berkeley was a distinguished Fellow of Trinity College and began writing philosophical works in his early 20s. His books included *An Essay Towards a New Theory of Vision* (1709), *Principles of Human Knowledge* (1710), and *Three Dialogues Between Hylas and Philonous* (1713).[38–40] His writings claimed that objects never observed by humans exist not because they are intrinsically "solid," but simply because God perceives them.[41,42]

Berkeley's views were complemented by those of another

idealist, the German philosopher George Wilhelm Friedrich Hegel (1770–1831). Hegel tried to construct a philosophy of "absolute idealism" in which the unfolding of the world over time reflected the majesty of God's mental growth.[43] As a young student at the University of Tübingen, Hegel had become drawn to mysticism, and he soon came to admire the grandness of self-appointed gods like Napoleon. Though he started his career as a private tutor in Bern and Frankfurt and served for a while as headmaster of a school in Nuremberg, Hegel's life evolved toward centers of power befitting a philosopher of the Cosmos. He completed his *Phenomenology of Mind* in Jena one day before a major battle occurred there. He became a professor in 1816 at Heidelberg and in 1818 at Berlin, where his interests and politics became aligned with the authoritarianism of the Prussian state. He died having made his "absolute idealism" the paramount philosophical ideal in Germany.[44–49]

Despite their initial appeal, purely mind-oriented notions like those of Berkeley and Hegel came to a bad end in the modern age. Popular sympathies eventually turned toward the theories of two other philosophers, David Hume and Immanuel Kant, whose writings undercut the theories of ontological idealists.

David Hume (1711–1776), a fiercely independent skeptic, was born in Edinburgh, Scotland. His father, owner of a small estate, died when he was an infant. Hume's mother urged him to obtain a law degree, but on admission to Edinburgh University at 12 years of age, he discovered that he craved only the study of philosophy and dropped out of school to study on his own. He made his living, after failing at a commercial venture in Bristol, as tutor to a Marquis, secretary to a general and a diplomat, and Librarian for the Faculty of Advocates in Edinburgh. His revolutionary monograph, the *Treatise of Human Nature*, upset almost every assumption of Western philosophy, though it found no audience when it was first published and failed to win Hume a faculty appointment at any university.[50–54]

Immanuel Kant (1724–1804), whose monumental system of philosophy Hume inspired, was born in Königsberg, East Prussia. His father, a religious pietist, worked as a humble saddler.

Kant spent his entire life in his home town, attended the local schools there, and ultimately found employment as a professor of logic and metaphysics at the University of Königsberg. His daily routine remained orderly and punctual throughout his life, which at first showed little hint of intellectual originality. Kant's early philosophical orientation stayed fairly close to the orthodoxies of his day, and his initial writings mainly concerned not metaphysics but the natural sciences. However, exposure to the skeptical works of Hume led him in the end to open new vistas for philosophy. Kant's major philosophical works included the *Critique of Pure Reason* (1781), *Prolegomena to Any Future Metaphysics* (1783), *Groundwork of the Metaphysic of Morals* (1785), *Critique of Practical Reason* (1788), and *Critique of Judgment* (1790).[55–60]

The thought of Hume and Kant is complex and will come up again later in this book. Most of its thrust is epistemological and ethical, not ontological. However, Hume and Kant did critically address the ontic idealism of Berkeley and, by implication, Hegel.

Berkeley and Hegel had based their theories on God's existence. Hume and Kant subverted this theistic assumption. Their reasoning showed that God's existence, even if real, cannot be proved logically.[61–63] The relevant arguments involved refuting the so-called "cosmological," "teleological," and especially "ontological" proofs of God's presence in the world.[64] Berkeley's idea of a material object as a concept in the mind of God and Hegel's notion of history as God's mental evolution could not survive such agnostic assaults. Hence, modern philosophy moved toward more secular foundations, damaging the idealists' program in its wake.

Meanwhile, "dualists" had come up with their own answers to the problems of ontology. They proposed a simultaneous co-existence for both mind and matter as separate realities. The French Renaissance thinker René Descartes (1596–1650), who is said to have invented modern philosophy, promoted such pluralistic views. Descartes' life overlapped those of other open minds like Fermat, Shakespeare, Milton, and Harvey. His speculative nature was fostered by supportive schooling at Poitiers and the Jesuit College of La Fléche, where the rector allowed him to lie in bed and think every morning. This practice afforded Descartes time to produce great intellectual insights. His expansive style further blossomed during his travels through Germany, Holland, and Italy after he had earned a law degree. In 1619, during a stay in Germany, Descartes experienced three dreams that inspired his entire subsequent philosophical outlook. He went on to produce a number of profound written works, including *Meditations on First Philosophy* (1641), *Rules for the Direction of Understanding* (1628), and *Discourse on Method* (1637). Descartes' productivity ceased only after 1649, when he moved to Sweden in order to tutor its queen; the monarch demanded severe working hours that took their toll on Descartes' frail constitution, terminated his habit of thinking in bed each morning, and led to his death from pneumonia within one year.[65–70]

Descartes' open-minded dualism transcended the restrictions of materialism and idealism. However, it also induced him to assert simplistically that the psyche and body interact through "pores" in the tiny pineal region of the brain. This claim seems odd today; its excessive concreteness points up a general defect in Descartes' ontology.

The flaw is this: Dualism requires that mind and matter interdependently influence each other[71–75] yet also maintain their status as ontological "substances," which are by definition independent. Such a concept of "psychosomatic" cause and effect makes no logical sense because it is self-contradictory. If we add to this problem Hume's insight that our perceptions of causality in general are more a "habit" of human thinking than anything inherent in nature,[76] ties between mind and matter become even more tenuous: Causality reveals itself as an unreliable avenue not only for mind–body links but also for relating any two classes of phenomena.

Gottfried Wilhelm von Leibnitz (1646–1716) accepted the coexistence of mind and matter but, unlike Descartes, tried to avoid the trap of a circularly causal nexus by denying the relevance of causation completely. Leibnitz came to such issues early in life. His father was a philosophy professor who gave his son's education a running start; Leibnitz was able to graduate from Leipzig University at the age of 16. He earned his law degree in 1666 at the University of Altdorf, declined a professorship there, and instead found work that sent him to Paris; there he encountered the "parallelist" philosopher Malebranche and the unpublished works of Descartes. When his employer died in 1673, Leibnitz became Librarian to the Electors of Brunswick in Hanover, reaching heights as a philosopher outside his job and in his spare time. His *Discourse on Metaphysics* and *Monadology* presented his views on relations between mind and matter. He explained semblances of cross talk between the brain and psyche as mere illusions, set up by a "preestablished harmony" between parallel mental and physical realms.[77–88]

Leibnitz's concepts were compelling, but they suffered ultimately from the same defects as those of Berkeley and Kant. Preestablishment of harmony between mind and matter could not be accomplished by mere mortals; it demanded a divine agent. Modern secular critics thus came to reject parallelism because of its dependence, like idealism, on religious premises.

Dualism in either its Cartesian or Leibnitzian guise has not solved the problem of mind–matter relations for modern philosophers. Cartesian views have turned out to be causally circular; Leibnitzian theories are theistically unprovable. As a result, dualism's agenda can only splinter into fruitless incoherence. Mind and matter seem to double back toward each other as mutually dependent negations and hence conflict as potentially inverse reductions of one another.[89] A dualist's groupings thus establish only relative links between mind and matter at any level of analysis.[90] Philosophers chasing an ever-receding goal of absolute dualism therefore become lost in an infinitely regressive wilderness of endlessly multiplying mind–body interfaces.[91–96]

Clearly, the best compromise between idealism and materialism to date does not lie in dualism. It lies instead in Baruch Spinoza's doctrine of neutral monism.[97–101]

Spinoza was unlike other philosophers of his day. He was born into the Jewish community of Amsterdam in 1632. His parents had emigrated there from the Iberian peninsula, where they had fled the Inquisition. Spinoza was raised and educated in the tradition of his faith, but also learned about secular thought from a Latin tutor, Van Den Ende. He developed heretical notions about the nature of God and sin, and his co-religionists took issue with these beliefs. Spinoza refused a bribe of 1000 florins to hide his ideas, survived a consequent assassination attempt, and was then ejected from the synagogue in 1656.

The liberal Dutch government, however, tolerated his opinions. Spinoza found the freedom to pursue friendships with members of the progressive Protestant sect called the Collegiants, who had no priests. He also took up lens grinding in order to earn a modest livelihood, though neither money nor marriage really interested him.

Spinoza's only true passion was philosophy. In his spartan bachelor's quarters in Amsterdam and then the Hague, Spinoza wrote responses to the problems created by dualism. He produced works that included the *Treatise on the Correction of the Understanding*, *Treatise on Politics*, *A Short Treatise on God, Man and his Well-Being*, *Tractatus Theologico-Politicus*, and his major opus, the *Ethics*. Spinoza's thought made him well known among the philosophers of his time, and he corresponded with many of them. However, he refused all offers of academic employment. In 1674, Christian authorities attacked and banned *Tractatus Theologico-Politicus*. Spinoza continued to write, but most of his manuscripts remained unpublished until after his death from tuberculosis in 1677 at the age of 43.[102–106]

Spinoza conceived the principles of neutral monism in order to better understand how apparent contrasts between mind and matter might hide an underlying connection. He suggested that mental and physical views of phenomena represent only divergent perspectives on the world. Reality, to which both subjective and objective languages ultimately refer, might seem either material or ideational, but such appearances depend only on the linguistic reference frames used to describe them. He thus postulated that the realms of mind and matter represent only differing facades conceived first under the [subjective] attribute of thought, secondly, under the [objective] attribute of [physical] extension.[107]

We can grasp this concept through the familiar fact that a conscious subject, encountering another conscious agent as object, does not simply act on the objective agent through cause and effect along a one-way street. The objective agent also acts from his own viewpoint as subject, setting his sights to transform the first subject into a material object. In this way, perceptions of conscious agents intertwine through changes in personal perspective.[108]

Spinoza suggested that a third "neutral" entity, comprising neither mind nor matter but appearing as either, lies prior to and beneath the changing illusion of subjective and objective viewpoints. This single "neutral" entity is the basic metaphysical substance sought since the days of Greek philosophers like Thales, Anaximenes, Heraclitus, Empedocles, Anaximander, and Plato. Such thinkers had all tried unsuccessfully to anchor their ideas about the world in a dependable, constant, intrinsic reality that would not change with the flux of appearances. Spinoza and subsequent neutral monists, including Hume, Russell, Strawson, and Feigl, continued the same search in a more modern idiom.[109–113]

The core attribute of any "neutral" and invariant reality is independence from the principle of causality.[114] Reference to causes and their effects usually reflects a need to bridge the gap opened by distinctions between knowing mental subjects and known physical objects.[115–119] We can close that gap, however, through a simple conceptual trick: We can exchange the role of subject and object in our imagination and thus identify invariant features through their survival, intact and unaltered, after the switch.

This maneuver is related to the idea of symmetry. Symmetry in mathematics describes any property that stays the same as other properties change. Mathematicians call the processes of change transformations and the items conserved, no matter what their character, invariants.

The idea of mathematical symmetry first became explicit through the struggles of Évariste Galois during the early 1800s. Galois was born in 1811 in the village of Bourg-la-Reine near Paris. His father was an antimonarchist politician who committed suicide after a scandal in 1829. Galois was tutored by his mother until the age of 12, when he entered school. He excelled in his academic studies and started his path-breaking research at the age of 16, but he became bored, and his conduct turned wild. At 17, he was unjustly rejected from the prestigious École Polytechnique for advanced mathematical training. He was denied recognition for his work throughout his lifetime, and his papers did not see the light of day until after his death. In frustration, Galois threw himself into revolutionary political activities, was arrested several times, and died in his 20th year on May 31, 1832, as the result of wounds sustained in a duel. However, through the medium of algebra, Galois left behind a rigorous conceptual basis for modern symmetry principles.[120,121]

Another great and more fortunate mathematician, Felix Klein (1849–1925), rooted symmetry in the geometric world by recasting geometric shapes as "groups" of symmetrical movements. Klein, like Galois, was intellectually precocious, but it also happened that his father was secretary to the Prussian *Regierungspräsident*. At 17, Klein gained the opportunity to work in an important physics laboratory in Bonn. By the age of 23, he had become a full professor of mathematics at Erlangen, married Hegel's granddaughter, and begun his masterwork, the Erlanger Programme. It was this project that recast all of geometry in terms of symmetries. Klein's gifts went on to grace a number of German universities, including those in Munich, Berlin, and Leipzig. His presence at Göttingen helped to make it a world center of mathematical learning.[122]

Klein's ideas created abstract notions of geometric symmetry that came to include not only the familiar mirror-like, left–right identity of shape implied in common parlance. This kind of "parity" invariance proved to represent only a single element among many other geometric symmetries.[123–127] Another example was "rotational" invariance, found, for instance, in the constant shape of a rigid globe as it turns on an axis. An even more exotic symmetry arose in the nonorientable two-dimensional space of a Möbius band. We can model this geometric construct as a long, rectangular strip of cellophane twisted in a one-half turn and then joined at its two ends. The image of an arrow, fastened to the strip and moved along its length, will change direction every time it completes a circuit through the strip. The arrow's flip-flop means that in global terms the Möbius band has only one assignable side. Its "sidedness" is invariant as the arrow moves.[128,129]

Mathematical concepts of symmetry have found their way into modern physics through formulations[130] even more generalizable than abstract geometric invariance. Symmetry has thus liberated modern physics from the classical straightjacket of over-concreteness and crude materialism. As pointed out by Nobel Prize laureate Richard Feynman,

> . . . it is not [simply] the symmetry of the [material] objects in nature that [is relevant] . . . here; it is rather the symmetry of the physical laws themselves. . . . [P]hysicists . . . have a feeling of symmetry about physical laws which is very close to the feeling of symmetry about objects. . . . [This is because] . . . there are things we can do to . . . our way of representing the physical laws, which make no difference, and leave everything unchanged in its effects.[131]

Symmetry can apply to subtle physical concepts, like the conservation of electrical charge, which have little direct relationship to ordinary Euclidean geometry or simple blobs of matter. Einstein provided the most famous example of a subtle physical symmetry, built on the ideas of Poincaré.[132] His invariant principle was the null influence of a moving body's speed on the laws governing electricity, magnetism, and the behavior of light signals in space and time. This kind of symmetry means that no physical communication using light can provide a yardstick or clock to distinguish one reference frame of motion from another. A strikingly counterintuitive result is the "twin paradox," which states that when one observer is traveling with respect to another fast enough to perceive time passing more slowly from his own perspective, the other observer also feels his own time passing more slowly.[133]

Anything, even if it is generalized above and beyond specific entities like Einstein's senders and receivers of light, can be seen as symmetrical; the only requirement for symmetry is that "there is something that you can do to it so that after you have finished doing it it looks the same as it did before."[134] Hence, we can invoke abstract analogies to physical symmetry when confronting broad philosophical issues like the mind–body problem and the metaphysical perspectives of neutral monism. It seems reasonable to explore the invariant "substance" envisioned by Spinoza as an entity that stays the same when subjective and objective reference frames change places.

In this kind of investigation we stand in good company. A few recent attempts to generalize new ideas from mathematical physics in order to relate mind and matter have approached the concept of symmetry per se. As one philosophically astute psychiatrist has observed, some contemporary thinkers are finally realizing that the outdated paradigms of classical physics impose "covert impediments to the development of new theories" even in psychology. Innovators have realized that alternative constructs abstracted from modern physics may illuminate areas untouched by old-fashioned mechanical dogmas.[135] Symmetry is the most potent among such modern concepts.

In fact, as we will see, parallels between symmetry in modern physics and neutral monism give us a tool to view the dismaying flaws inherent in neuropsychiatry as mere conceptual limits and hence find ways beyond them. This is so because neutral monism is not simply the one philosophical alternative to materialism that modern neuropsychiatrists can accept[136,137]; it also constitutes a platform from which to look for a more comprehensive philosophy of mind. The symmetry properties of neutral monism therefore merit our further attention. A particular aspect of their importance is a connection to concepts of numerical measurement in neuroscience.

4

Neuropsychiatry and Numbers

Neuropsychiatrists confer a seeming validity on their ideas by linking them to numbers. The brain itself has been selected as an object of study because of its measurable dimensions: length, width, depth, weight, motion, temperature, and electrical charge. Indeed, the rising tide of neuropsychiatry might be best understood as little more than a search for one-to-one numerical correlations between mental symptoms and abnormalities within the brain. In this way, biological psychiatry tries to conform to demands of technical science for objectivity and quantitative exactitude.[1]

Number worship of the sort common among neuroscientists goes all the way back to Pythagoras, who is said to have been born on the Greek isle of Samos near the coast of Ionia in about 570 BC. The details of his life are sketchy, having come down to us through subsequent philosophers such as Plato, Aristotle, and Dicaearchus, but some facts are known. Pythagoras apparently fled Samos in order to escape the tyrant Polycrates. He traveled through Egypt, where he picked up concepts of numerology. He also passed through Babylonia; there he encountered and embraced many native algebraic notions, though he resisted the practical orientation of Babylonian culture in favor of pure mathematical theory and philosophy.

Pythagoras settled in Crotona, a Greek colony of about

300,000 people located in the southern Italian region of Magna Graecia, and lectured widely about mathematics. He formed a group, the Pythagorean Society, devoted to the study of mathematics, astronomy, and music, and married one of his students. Over time, the group became a secretive order. Its members sought to move beyond the empirical basis of Egyptian and Babylonian ideas about numbers to a more logically rigorous style, borrowed from Pythagoras' predecessor, Thales. The resulting method of deductive proof started with a bare minimum of basic assumptions, or axioms, and derived all other principles of mathematics as theorems stemming from those axioms. The technique was refined by subsequent Greek thinkers until it reached maturity in the thought of Euclid about two centuries after Pythagoras' death.

The Pythagorean Society sought patterns in the behavior of numbers. Toward this end, it investigated the behavior of triangles, rectangles, pentagons, and other regular geometric figures with regard to the lengths of their sides. In line with such "figurative" thinking, the Pythagoreans came to picture numbers divisible by two as rectangular arrays of dots distributed in even numbers of columns. Odd numbers were similar, except that to each array one additional dot was added.

This tidy way of tracking numbers might by itself appear somewhat prosaic. However, Pythagorean concerns went beyond mere logical proof, figurative analogy, geometric exactitude, and empirical observation; interests extended into the realm of mysticism. This "akousmatic" outlook was thoroughgoing and all-pervasive. Pythagoras' followers prayed at least as much as they deliberated. Disciples eschewed the eating of animal flesh and beans. Their eclectic and bizarre ritual laws forbade stirring fires with iron instruments, walking on highways, looking into mirrors that stood next to lights, plucking garlands, stepping over crossbars, laughing excessively, and allowing swallows to live on the roofs of homes. The faithful also believed in the transmigration of souls, which they called "metempsychosis."

Mysticism suffused Pythagorean numerical concepts. Pythagoras saw in each number a unique, symbolic meaning. The number 4, for example, embodied justice; 3 represented men; 2 stood for women. The numeral 1 symbolized reason, but it was not quite considered a real number, since its use required no act of counting; Pythagoras regarded the notion of unity as only a "source" for numerical concepts.

Classes and agglomerations of numbers also took on mystical significance. The even numbers were considered feminine, the odd numbers masculine. The "tetraktys of the decad," an equilateral triangle of ten dots with four dots on each side and one in the center, became Pythagoras' basis for the whole physical world. He used it as "evidence" for four universal elements: earth, fire, air, and water.

Pythagoreans adhered to their leader's maxim that numbers rather than material substances govern the universe, thus determining the content not of only mathematics but also of the natural sciences. This "cosmogony" led to a distinction between integers, used for counting, and real numbers, employed for measurement. It also created a conceptual crisis.

From square arrays of dots, the Pythagoreans were able to visualize the concept of an integer multiplied by itself. Investigations of musical overtones led to the idea of dividing integers into harmonic ratios that involve fractions. Crisis arose when concepts of squared integers led Pythagoras to see that ratios between measurable lengths assigned to the hypotenuse and one side of a right triangle may not be calculable in a finite number of steps. This threw the Pythagorean faith that "numbers and their ratios rule the universe" into doubt. It showed that countable integers and measurable numbers are "incommensurable."

One might think of commensurability in terms of shoes in a closet: If all shoes are members of a matched pair, then the number of left shoes and the number of right shoes reflects a one-to-one correspondence between left and right shoes. Incommensurable objects like integers and "real" numbers cannot be placed in one-to-one correspondence with each other without some real numbers being left over at the end of the hypothetical matching process.[2–8]

One-to-one correspondence figures prominently in the definition of number given by three important modern philosophers of mathematics[9]: Gottlob Frege, Alfred North Whitehead, and Bertrand Russell.

Frege, the senior member of the trio, was born in 1848. He wrote unobtrusively at the University of Jena for 30 years until his death in 1925 and came by his insights without any ongoing collaboration. Frege's *Foundations of Arithmetic* and other works created the basis for twentieth-century mathematical logic, although his importance was not appreciated until well after he died.[10–12]

Whitehead, the next member of the trio, was born in 1861 in London. His student days were spent at Sherborne and Trinity College. Whitehead first established himself as a mathematician in Cambridge and London, then as a philosopher at Harvard. His outlook was largely empirical. He worked with Russell in an attempt to reduce all mathematics to logic; the result was their famous book, *Principia Mathematica*. Whitehead also singly authored several other books, including *Principles of Natural Knowledge*, *The Concept of Nature*, *Science and the Modern World*, *Process and Reality*, and *Adventures of Ideas*. He died in 1947.[13,14]

Russell was born in 1872 to an upper-class English family and studied mathematics and philosophy at Cambridge. A conversation with the Italian mathematician Peano at a Paris conference led Russell to join Whitehead in their *Principia* project. Thereafter, Russell became embroiled in political activities, including an unsuccessful bid for a seat in Parliament and outspoken efforts on behalf of pacifism, women's suffrage, and agnosticism. His political positions led to a brief jail sentence in 1918, during which he wrote the *Introduction to Mathematical Philosophy*. After his release from prison, Russell's career and personal life became even more volatile. Nonetheless, he produced copious writings and in 1944 was offered the status of Fellow at Trinity College. Russell moved to North Wales in 1955 and again became outspoken in politics, eventually condemning both American conduct in Vietnam and Israeli actions in the 1967 Middle East War. He remained intellectually conspicuous until his death at the age of 98.[15-17]

Frege, Whitehead, and Russell all portrayed numbers as self-contained, independent invariants that stay the same under circumstances in which elements of different categories can be exchanged in a one-to-one manner. The idea may be understood by returning to the image of shoes in a closet. If all shoes are members of a matched pair, then not only do the left and right shoes demonstrate a one-to-one correspondence; the number of left shoes, right shoes, and *pairs* of shoes are all commensurable. The number of objects in a subordinate category such as left shoes thus emerges as the superordinate entity germane to all categories, whose constituent objects are in one-to-one correspondence with those of the given category. The superordinate numerical entity remains invariant no matter which subcategory of equinumerous objects is counted.

This invariance plays into the Pythagorean agenda by elevating pure numbers to the symmetrical status of a "substance."[18] It also relates to the role of neutral monism in providing a quantitative foundation for neuropsychiatry.[19,20] The invariant "substance" postulated by neutral monism exhibits symmetry insofar as it remains the same when subjects and objects exchange roles in a commensurable, one-to-one manner; numbers arise naturally in this one-to-one exchange. Hence, number reveals itself as the invariant property of neutral monism in support of the view that mathematics can provide the key to understanding our universe.[21]

The idea of numbers as the basis of all reality has found especially receptive ears in recent times. The concept took root at the beginning of the twentieth century, when three rival schools of thought about numbers were battling for dominance in the world of mathematics. These schools were called intuitionism, logicism, and formalism.

E. J. Brouwer (1881–1966), a Dutch mathematics professor, founded the intuitionist school of mathematics on the basis of ideas put forward by such predecessors as Kronecker, Borel, Lebesgue, Poincaré, and Baire.[22] His followers attempted to remove concepts of infinity from mathematical discourse, but mathematicians could not accept this crippling limit on their creative resources.

The logicists, including Frege and Russell, tried to base mathematics on logical truth alone. However, paradoxes arose in the very fabric of their project. These torpedoed much of the movement.

Therefore, by default, the formalists won out. They were spearheaded by David Hilbert (1862–1943). Hilbert had come from a distinguished German family and earned his doctorate in 1884 at the University of Königsberg. At the urging of Felix Klein, Hilbert joined the Göttingen faculty in 1895 and worked there until his retirement in 1930. Among his many achievements, Hilbert provided an axiomatic foundation for the formalist program, which judged mathematical theories by their internal self-consistency.[23]

After Hilbert passed from the scene, however, formalism degenerated into a view of mathematics as mere symbol-juggling. It dismissed as irrelevant the tangible objects to which numerals refer. Rigid proponents of formalistic proof thus came to prefer "pure," self-referent mathematics over activities applied to content-laden areas, which it arbitrarily exiled from its own domain and demoted in prestige.[24,25] Consequently, mathematical formalism not only skewed its own priorities but also biased the empirical quantitative sciences toward worship of counting and measurement as primary methods of inquiry. Formalism's marriage with metaphysics hence fueled our modern need to ground all forms of scientific scholarship in numbers.

During the Renaissance, the great Italian physicist Galileo Galilei (1564–1642) had planted his own seeds for this kind of prejudice. He characterized proper science as involving only quantitative concepts.[26] This view carried weight because Galileo had virtually created modern empirical physics. After defying his father's wishes for him to pursue other lines of study, Galileo attended the University of Pisa, became a mathematician in the court of Florence, and taught at several universities. He then formulated theories about the motion of projectiles and innovatively tested them through precise experiments. Galileo's endorsement of heretical ideas earned him the wrath of the Catholic Church and a life sentence of house arrest.[27] Yet his groundbreaking research techniques left him without any doubt that "the book of nature is written in the language of mathematics."[28]

Ernst Mach, a late nineteenth-century philosopher of physics whose interests spilled into many other areas of inquiry, pushed Galileo's approach to its limits as a modern obsession. Mach had been born in Moravia and taught mathematics at Graz. He acquired an early respect for empirical data-gathering, making a name for himself in gas flow research. By the year 1900, he had become professor of physics in Prague and then Vienna. At that time, his thoughts returned to a philosophical vision from his youth.

Mach had become convinced of his own illusory nature as a qualitative "self."[29,30] This led him to seek refuge in a view of science as a purely quantitative affair. He rejected the relevance of all personally "preconceived" speculations. Only events that could be measured experimentally won any place in his system of thought. Other concepts lost their claim to independent meaning and became solely ways of relating experimental data themselves.

Mach died in 1916. His subordination of speculative theory to quantitative experiment spurred the new philosophical school of logical positivism. Several of the original positivists came from quantitative backgrounds like Mach's. Philipp Frank, for example, was a physicist. Rudolph Carnap had begun a doctoral program in physics before World War I interrupted his studies. Moritz Schlick had learned physics at the University of Berlin under the great Max Planck. Gustav Bergmann, Hans Hahn, Karl Menger, and Kurt Reidemeister were all mathematicians. Together, these men and others formed the famous Vienna Circle.[31,32]

The group's fundamental "principle of verification" engrafted Mach's ideas onto the formal algebra of logic conceived by Frege, Russell, Whitehead, Leibnitz, Boole, de Morgan, and Peano.[33,34]

The principle asserted that no utterance, by a physicist or anyone else, has scientific validity unless it can be precisely measured against experience. The doctrine excluded more ethereal, qualitative assertions from all debate. Statements concerning ethics, for example, became candidates for the scrap heap.[35]

In 1927, Percy Bridgeman (1882–1961) took positivistic ideas even further. Bridgeman was trained as a physicist, did research at Harvard on the electrical and thermal characteristics of matter under high pressure, and won a Nobel Prize for his work. He formulated a view of science known as operationalism, explicated in books like his *Logic of Modern Physics* (1927). Bridgeman's doctrines asserted that the numerical data of science have little to do even with the facts of an independent physical reality. The sole meaning of a scientific statement lay not in passive perceptions of an objective universe; it lay instead in equations that a scientist conceives for purposes of active experimental measurement. Bridgeman saw nothing in his scientific craft beyond concepts of a yardstick, thermometer, scale, or clock.[36,37]

The positivism of the Vienna Circle and the operationalism of Bridgeman extended the numerical biases of physical measurement into every field of study. Psychology was not exempt.[38–40] Its practitioners launched attempts to force all psychological language into a measurable mold.[41–43] Quantitative psychologists were following Mach's own lead in this project: Mach's books had included titles like *The Analysis of the Sensations* and *The Relation of the Physical to the Psychical*.

Mathematical methods of classical physics seduced a large following of psychologists and psychiatrists. The prior success of measurement in explaining inanimate processes and harnessing them into useful technology inspired many students of the mind to borrow the most potent procedures of physical science for their own areas of inquiry. In this spirit, they aimed to abolish all qualitative "speculation" about the mind and replace it with pure numerical data.[44]

Early practical expressions of the movement to turn mind into quantifiable data appeared during the nineteenth century. In 1846,

Ernst Weber (1795–1878), a professor of anatomy and physiology in Leipzig[45] and the first rigorous experimental researcher in psychology, invented a quantitative laboratory paradigm which he called his "just noticeable differences" law. The principle connected objective stimulus magnitudes with the subjective human ability to perceive discrepancies between stimuli.

Gustav Fechner (1801–1887) extended Weber's quantitative experimental approach. Fechner came to his work armed with a background combining a medical degree and a faculty appointment in the physics department of Leipzig University. He exploited Weber's techniques in order to establish a psychophysical scale of metric units with a zero point. He also adapted probability theory to his experimental efforts, producing methods that represented the beginning of quantitative statistical work in the psychological laboratory.[46] Fechner's aim was the merger of psychology and physics into a new discipline whose name formed part of the title given to his 1860 book, *Elements of Psychophysics*.[47,48]

Hermann von Helmholtz (1821–1894) studied life processes, including those of the mind, with even stricter experimental measurement. He began his career as a physiologist, serving on the faculties of universities in Königsberg, Bonn, and Heidelberg; during this time, in 1858, he successfully measured the speed at which an electrical impulse travels along a nerve fiber. Helmholtz's achievements multiplied and spilled over into other areas of science; he originated the quantitative principle of energy conservation using data derived from animal experiments and earned a professorship in physics at the University of Berlin in 1871. Helmholtz also invented new technical tools like the ophthalmoscope, ophthalmometer, acoustic resonator, and tachistoscope. He thus enhanced the precision of psychophysical experiments and was able to measure such perceptual phenomena as blind spots, afterimages, chromatic aberration, venous shadows, and combination tones. His writings included the *Treatise on Physiological Optics* and *On the Sensations of Tone*.[49,50]

Wilhelm Wundt (1832–1920) expanded the quantitative work of Weber, Fechner, and Helmholtz. Wundt had attended school at

Tübingen and studied physiology in Berlin. He went on to obtain a medical degree at the University of Heidelberg, where the influence of Helmholtz as chairman could be felt. Wundt developed his outlook on the mind in Heidelberg and wrote his book, *Principles of Physiological Psychology*, there. He then moved to Leipzig, where as professor he started the world's first experimental psychology laboratory. His psychophysical research program, like those of Weber, Fechner, and Helmholtz, aimed at measuring sensory responses to tightly controlled physical stimuli. An elite group of expert subjects, trained to estimate the numerical intensity of their own sensations, provided Wundt's data. He strove for maximal precision in designing his studies.[51,52]

Students who had flocked to Wundt's laboratory extended his quantitative methods to exotic domains of inquiry. Several English and American protégés returned to their own countries and spread a new, universal gospel of mental measurement.[53]

Extreme fringes of the empirical movement, trying for the sake of objectivity to banish even notions of sensation from psychology, coalesced in the "behaviorist" work of John Broadus Watson. His concepts stemmed partly from Wundt's disciples and partly from the work of Russian reflexologists Bekhterev, Sechenov, and Pavlov.

Watson was born near Greenville, South Carolina, in 1878. He grew up in impoverished rural circumstances, attended a local college, and then earned a Ph.D. in psychology at the University of Chicago under James Rowland Angell, John Dewcy, H. H. Donaldson, and Jaques Loeb. Watson went on to direct the psychology laboratory at the University of Chicago and then accepted a post at Johns Hopkins, where he became chairman of the psychology department.

In 1913, Watson established the principles of behaviorism in a lecture entitled "Psychology as the Behaviorist Views It." He also proclaimed his ideas and methods in four books, published from 1913 to 1928. He saw behavioral science as totally objective; in his eyes, there was no room for subjective, sensory concepts or introspection. The very design of his experiments, concentrating only on motor behavior, afforded subjects little chance to infect objective behavioral measurements with subjective contaminants.

By 1915, such concepts had propelled Watson to the presidency of the American Psychological Association. Four years later Watson was applying his ideas, originally culled from work with rats, to human infants. However, a personal scandal drove him from the faculty at Johns Hopkins in 1920, after which he worked in the advertising industry. He died in 1958.[54–58]

Despite his early departure from academics, Watson's outlook attracted many other psychologists in the 1930s and 1940s. One colleague in the behaviorist camp was Clark L. Hull (1884–1952) of Yale University, who had planned to become an engineer until illness thwarted his goals. His interest in numbers found an outlet in attempts to create a purely theoretical superstructure for psychology akin to the system of axioms invented for arithmetic by mathematical formalists. In the 1950s, Hull's ideas gradually gave way to those of yet other behaviorists, who also embraced only quantifiable phenomena.[59–61]

Meanwhile, numerical scoring of personality traits took root with Jung's Word Association Test in 1918, Rorschach's famous inkblots in 1921, Hathaway and McKinley's Minnesota Multiphasic Personality Inventory (MMPI) in 1943, and Millon's Clinical Multiaxial Inventory in the 1980s. David Wechsler, working at Bellevue in 1939, created a new quantitative yardstick for the intellect in the form of his Wechsler–Bellevue Scale, which evolved into the Wechsler Adult Intelligence Scale (WAIS) in 1955 and the WAIS-R in 1981.[62]

Metric psychology thus emerged to drive psychological researchers on toward greater and greater numerical precision in their experimental measurements. It served as a modern conduit for the number worship inherent in the Pythagorean tradition, turn-of-the-century mathematics, logical positivism, German psychophysics, American behaviorism, and several versions of neutral monism. Metric psychology hence provided a model for medically oriented neuropsychiatry, with its penchant for clinical data honed to the last possible decimal place.[63]

5

Computers and the Mind

R ecently, metric psychology and its parent, neutral monism, have begun to encourage "functionalist" approaches to the mind. These liken the mental processes of living, sentient organisms to the workings of a machine.[1]

The influence of neutral monism is easily seen in such analogies. Programmable "functions" of a machine are neither subjective mind nor matter, but something else again. They are objective yet harbor an abstract structure that is independent of the material hardware supporting them.[23] This latter fact has allowed functionalists to choose arbitrarily among all kinds of machine metaphors, including those of a catapult, mill, hydraulic lift, weaver's loom, telegraph, and phone switchboard, in discussing the mind's ostensible "design."

Functional analogies between machines and minds have spawned the supreme numerical bias in psychology. These metaphors cast the mind as a computer.

Computational data processing numerically encodes not only arithmetical but also other components of its programs.[4,5] Therefore, computers might be seen in terms of quantities that relate to each other in the style of a self-contained symmetry.[6] The use of numbers to express computer language hence exhibits invariance when subjective and objective reference frames undergo one-to-one exchanges. Computer-oriented cognitive science and artificial intelligence theories thus implicitly seem to embrace the neutrally monistic symmetry of self-referent numbers.

The image of our mind as a computing mechanism has caught on. It fires the imagination of not only professionals but also the general public through popular media. One TV documentary on brain science, for instance, describes what lies within the human head as "the guts of the most complex machine in the world." Robert Heinlein's science fiction novel, *The Moon Is a Harsh Mistress*, paints the convincing portrait of a computer that achieves brainlike consciousness.[7]

Though functionalists see the brain as only one of many possible computer hardwares that might subserve mental processes,[8–10] they look to brain architecture as the actual embodiment of our own human minds in nature. The billions of working cells[11] located in the brain are now widely deemed to behave as discrete and countable microunits. Many functionalists have therefore felt justified in assigning to brains a "digital" computer design, which for its ability to calculate relies on discrete components that can be added, subtracted, multiplied, and divided.[12] Were the brain to consist of a continuous fiber network without any gaps between units of nerve tissue as was once believed,[13] the whole digital computer metaphor would be thrown into disarray. But the contemporary digital model of microscopic brain organization draws apparent support from a long series of empirical observations.

In 1811, Charles Bell distinguished between distinct motor and sensory nerve "fibers." Francois Magendie showed in 1822 that sensory nerves enter and motor fibers exit the spinal cord at separate locations. Magendie's structural work heralded subsequent "atomic" behavioral concepts of the discrete reflex arc, developed by Marshall Hall in 1833, embellished by David Hartley, and later applied to the brain and behavior by Laycock, Sechenov, Bekhterev, and Pavlov.[14]

Meanwhile, Franz Joseph Gall (1758–1828) discovered that, besides the white matter comprising all fibrous neural material, the nervous system also contains gray matter. This gray matter includes brain cell "bodies," like those later discovered by Meynert, Betz, Campbell, and Brodmann on the surface or "cortex" of the brain. In 1849, Rudolph Von Kolliker linked fibers and cell bodies into units, later dubbed "neurons" by Waldeyer.[15]

In 1873, Camillo Golgi (1843–1926), professor of pathology at Pavia, made a critical research breakthrough by pioneering the use of a microscopic silver chromate dye that picks out single units at random from hundreds in a given network.[16,17] This staining technique allowed the Spanish histologist Santiago Ramón y Cajal (1852–1934) to identify individual neurons among the many packed together so densely in the brain that they could not otherwise be distinguished. Ramón y Cajal confirmed that every neuron consists of a main clump of material, the body, as well as fibrous fingers, called axons and dendrites, that extend toward other neurons. He found that each axon, as it approaches another cell, ends in an enlarged, bulbous segment. He shared the Nobel Prize for this work with Golgi.[18]

Ramón y Cajal postulated that a gap lies between any axon terminal and the next neuron. In 1897, Sir Charles Sherrington (1857–1952), another eminent neuroscientist, endorsed the idea of these gaps and named them synapses. Sherrington's support carried prestige because of his own outstanding independent achievements. He had been born in London, attended Cambridge, trained as a physician at St. Thomas' Hospital in London, and become a professor at Oxford. He was made a fellow of the Royal Society and won the Nobel prize in 1932. His best-known published work was *The Integrative Action of the Nervous System* of 1908, but his writings also included *Mammalian Physiology*, *Reflex Activity in the Spinal Cord*, several other books, and over 300 technical papers. His studies of primitive brain reflexes in animals, their integration at higher levels of brain function, and their survival value for the organism combined the precision of experimental neuroscience with the imagination of a philosopher.[19,20] His enthusiasm for synaptic concepts therefore lent them weight.

Synapses were ultimately visualized by electron microscopy,[21] and this evidence led to a general acceptance by virtually all neuroscientists. The digital concept of neurons as discrete, individual cells in the brain thus became a familiar part of the landscape for researchers, who incorporated the idea into their manifold explorations of neuronal chemistry, structure, and especially electrical properties.

The discovery of electrical potentials in individual neurons led researchers to ask questions about the brain as a mass of digital circuits. Galvani in 1780 linked electricity to the twitching of a frog's leg. In 1848, Du Bois Reymond[22] demonstrated a difference in voltage between the injured and intact ends of isolated fibers. Bernstein in 1866 showed that the intrinsic activity of nervous tissue is electrical in nature.[23]

Workers subsequently began to analyze the ability of neurons to respond with electrical discharges of their own when irritated by an outside voltage source. They found that if a unit anywhere in the nervous system receives more than a small amount of energy from an experimental electrode, it reacts by firing a volley of self-generated electrical bursts, called "action potentials." The combined research of three different neurophysiologists, Richard Caton, Hans Berger, and Edgar Adrian, demonstrated spontaneous electrical phenomena produced by neurons specifically located within the brain.[24] Caton, a young assistant in physiology at the Liverpool Royal Infirmary, discovered the EEG in animals in 1875.[25,26] Berger's work in Jena during the 1920s and 1930s produced the first human electroencephalographic recording.[27,28] Adrian's research at Cambridge confirmed Berger's findings.[29,30]

Dr. Mary Brazier of UCLA summarized electrophysiology's pivotal role in probing the brain's computerlike operating "codes." She wrote that

> the single most important discovery in the exploration of nervous mechanisms was that the nerve impulse is identical with an electrical change. This electrical sign of activity has given the investigator a means of studying the functioning nervous system—a tracer by which he can

follow impulses in the living organism through the complexity of structure that the microscope can only reveal in dead tissue. It is also the only clue he has as to how messages may be coded in the nervous system.[31]

However, some vehicle other than the internally generated electrical activity of single neurons was required to bridge the external jump across intercellular "synaptic" gaps.[32] Loewi showed in 1921 that chemical intermediaries perform this task. In 1936, Dale identified one of those "transmitter" chemicals as acetylcholine. Other analogous substances such as dopamine, norepinephrine, and serotonin emerged in later work.[33]

It was found empirically that neurons squirt these chemicals into synapses. The unloosed transmitter molecules flow toward an adjacent cell on the other side of each gap, contact its receptor membranes, and influence its electrical charge. As Sherrington suggested in 1906, chemical signals thus allow brain cells to exert both excitatory and inhibitory influences on each other. If in response to transmitter chemicals a postsynaptic charge changes enough and in the proper direction, action potentials spring up in the receptor cell. If charges move in the opposite direction, receptor action potentials are suppressed.

In the view of many scientists, synaptic gaps and the molecular messengers floating within them hence began to appear as perfect sites for the computerlike integration of digital electrical "software" coding in brain cells. Researchers created tools to study both healthy and pathological intercellular hookups. One new type of chemical pigment was developed by Walle Nauta, a prominent investigator working near Washington, DC, and at the Massachusetts Institute of Technology. His technique highlighted only fibers emanating from dying cell bodies, so that brain structures of experimental animals could reveal their projections to distant synapses after deliberate, focused damage in the laboratory. Radiation detectors, through "hot" travels of injected tracer elements, also mapped the far reaches of an axon. Enzymes, antibodies, and many other tools entered the synaptologist's trade.[34,35]

Two methods of inquiry have received special attention in recent years. One applies to small groups of cells and the other works on a larger scale, but both are said to carry implications about the role of synapses in mental processes.

At a microscopic level, work on the physiology of learning in simple animals has identified assemblies of linked neurons whose electrochemical junctions change as behavior shifts.[36] These results have led to conclusions that explain some types of memory in terms of synaptic mechanisms.

At the macroscopic level, interplay between masses of nerve cells has become evident through the use of PET and SPECT machines. Scientists connect different neuron populations by correlating their sugar consumption or blood flow rates. On the basis of such data, activation of tissue both near the brain's surface and in deeper regions by visual stimuli has been attributed to axonal links. Some researchers have tried relating these findings to behavior, mood, intellectual activity, and mental disturbances.[37,38]

Efforts to find new tools for probing the connections between brain cells are always under way. Investigators have sought the means to inhibit all neurons of only a single type and to stain neurons adjacent to a dye-injected cell through synaptic contacts. Scientists are also working for better ways to record the electrical activity of many brain cells simultaneously.[39]

The concept of brain hardware or "wetware," which embodies and supports mental software, thus has found wide acceptance. The role of electrical conduits has fallen to brain cells and that of switches to intervening synapses. The model seems to make some sense in light of repeated observations that intelligent animals with the greatest "computational power" possess richer links among more cells than do primitive creatures.[40] Hence, many scientists hope to match normal behavior in humans with specific connections among neurons.

Neuropsychiatrists, either implicitly or explicitly, incorporate this kind of analogy into their own outlook. They are prone to see the thinking brain as a "very large network of different communication centers that can flash on and off and send messages to one another through electrical impulses."[41] They assume that "when we talk, think, feel, or dream, each of these mental functions is due to . . . circuits that make up the human brain."[42]

Moreover, almost all contemporary theories about the neural causes of mental illness can be translated into a species of analogy to bad wiring, portraying psychological pain as "neurophysiological glitches."[43] To the extent that researchers view nerve fibers as cablelike structures and their transmitter substances as switching mechanisms, neuropsychiatric ideas about disease must bear at least some kinship to the notion of a damaged logic board or chip. Neuropsychiatrists tend to endorse such a view of psychiatric disease as "disruptions in the normal flow of messages through . . . [brain] circuitry"[44] due to a "fault" in the "pattern of wiring," in the "command centers," or in the "way messages move along the wires."[45]

The functionalistic image of a deranged mind as a broken computing mechanism has reached the public in force. Many popular science fiction movies feature gadgets that become mentally ill. In some of these films men and machines become locked in combat to determine whether the wetware of the brain or the hardware of computers will prove more fit for survival. There is a natural progression from this kind of fearful speculation to the theories of sociobiology.

Sociobiologists assert that behavioral imperatives, including those of "higher" morality, arise from the strict mathematical laws of genetics, subject to selection by the Darwinian demands of survival and biological reproduction. Sociobiologists thus advocate locating the ultimate evolutionary sources of behavioral motivation, including the "software" that "directs the assembly" of neuronal networks, in DNA sequences contained by genes throughout all the body's cells. This view seems plausible insofar as DNA's bare, ribbonlike molecular appearance and mechanical language resemble the conceptual precursors of all modern computers, Turing machines.[46-50]

The theoretical outlook implicit in sociobiology has found practical expression in the complementary research paradigms of ethology,[51] which studies innate behaviors in the wild, and psychogenetics,[52] which emphasizes statistical measurement. But more importantly, linkage between behavior and the computable aspects of genetics has spawned a specific control-systems approach to the evolution of the brain. In the late nineteenth and early twentieth centuries, two scientists, Conwy Lloyd Morgan and John Hughlings Jackson, hinted at this in their analyses of behavior as a hierarchy of emergent properties evolving from simpler, automatic mechanisms into more complex entities associated with "higher" consciousness.[53]

Lloyd Morgan, born in London in 1852, was the less clinically oriented of the two. He enrolled at the School of Mines and Royal College of Science, planning to become a mining engineer, but a mentor, T. H. Huxley, prevailed upon him to turn toward the study of instinctual behavior among animals. Lloyd Morgan spent five years in South Africa and in 1884 became professor of geology and zoology at the University College of Bristol, where he rose in rank to the position of vice-chancellor. His concept of trial-and-error learning became widely influential. In honor of accomplishments including two important books, *Animal Life and Intelligence* and *An Introduction to Comparative Anatomy*, he became the first psychologist elected to the Royal Society. He retired in 1919 and died in 1936.[54]

Lloyd Morgan addressed the issue of control systems in the brain by asserting that higher centers can exert influence by either augmenting or inhibiting primitive components of the nervous system. In decoding emergent loci of behavior, Lloyd Morgan invoked his methodological "canon" of parsimony, a kind of psychological Occam's Razor requiring that any observed behavior be interpreted as output from the lowest and simplest organizational level consistent with relevant empirical phenomena.[55]

John Hughlings Jackson (1835–1911), now considered by many to be the father of British neurology, translated such ideas into his own concept of vertically emergent brain organization. Jackson worked in London as a physician at the National Hospital for Nervous Diseases, Queen Square, where he achieved eminence in many areas of neurology. During his career, Jackson had successfully inferred functional neuroanatomy of the brain from the progression of events occurring during epileptic attacks. He also had correctly understood aphasia as a disorder of language rather than of simple mechanical speech and had made the suggestion, years ahead of its time, that spatial abilities are a function of the right half of the brain. Jackson solidified theories of emergent brain evolution by suggesting that neural tissue is organized into three distinct levels. These, in ascending order, are the "lower" reflex pathways, "middle" centers, and consciously volitional "higher" structures. Jackson also streamlined existing ideas about emergence by jettisoning the concept of augmenting mechanisms and suggesting that higher structures control and coordinate lower centers mainly through inhibition. He speculated that damage to vulnerable higher brain centers expresses itself pathologically as release of hardier lower functions.[56]

These ideas make the notion of a neural "drive center," linking higher brain regions to the lower centers that they control, appear to be a sound and worthwhile concept today. The "lower" areas of the human brain are identified as those that regulate the body's internal equilibrium; "higher" regions ostensibly direct interaction with the external world. It thus seems only reasonable to argue that an intermediate "drive center," by breaching rationally apportioned boundaries between the body's interior and exterior, actually subserves the illogical processes of the passions.[57,58] Tempting evidence for this view arises in experimentally observed mixing of physiological signals related to contradictory motivational drives. The effects of stimulation in one part of the ostensible "drive center" have been observed to spill over into adjacent parts and thus evoke additional, often conflicting emotions.

Neuropsychiatric ideas about mental illness fit well with this kind of model. The concept of "schizophysiology," originally advanced by Paul D. MacLean of the Laboratory for Brain Evolution and Behavior at the National Institute of Mental Health,[59] suggests that irrational aspects of human mental illness derive from imperfect control of primitive brain centers by higher structures. Efficient control of these primitive mechanisms by higher brain functions may not yet have had time to evolve completely in "schizophysiological" humans. The resulting imperfections might sometimes release passions of the beast when logic should prevail. Such theories have gained a wide following throughout the scientific community.[60-64]

Images of control, both efficient and imperfect, have proliferated to affect understanding of brain architecture even beyond its evolutionary aspects. Several famous biologists have helped to give the idea of brain control systems a prominent overall place in neuroscience.

Claude Bernard (1813–1878), a seminal figure in modern experimental physiology, began the trend in the 1850s. Bernard had worked as a druggist's assistant and made a failed attempt at a literary career before enrolling in medical school and finally becoming a professor at the College de France. His wide-ranging physiological research brought him world fame. Bernard made a strong case for his idea that the visceral nervous system automatically monitors, controls, and hence maintains constancy of the body's internal environment. He suggested that this is accomplished by feedback loops wired to neural reflex arcs.[65]

In 1928, Walter B. Cannon (1871–1945) extended this notion to the emotions, which he claimed are regulated by selected circuits in the brain.[66] Cannon, born in Wisconsin, attended Harvard, where he became a professor at the medical school. His work began with research on the act of swallowing, but eventually he branched out into other visceral mechanisms and their relationship to emotions. In the process of conducting his studies, Cannon conceived the idea of "homeostasis," which mathematicians subsequently developed into a formal feedback theory of servocontrol in cybernetic devices.[67] Cannon's concept in its more general mathematical form enabled investigators like Miller, Galanter, and Pribram in 1960 to draw analogies between an organism's plan for living and the sequence control of a computer program.[68]

Current proponents of control schemes liken emotional life to a feedback system between endocrine glands or similar target organs and the brain. They understand related neural structures as "filters" feeding data back to the cortex for selective perception and memory storage.[69–71] They even try to locate control of all conscious states in a command module at the brain's anatomical core.[72,73]

There is a good reason for these recurrent images of control in functional neuroscience. The coordinating hallmark not only of genes and computerlike "brains" but also of all computer systems in practical use today is a control module in the form of a central processing unit. The control module oversees the workings of all other parts from the "top down" by overarching principles extending to specific cases.[74]

This is the reason that notions of a central command center have flourished in computer models of mind and brain. It has led modern experimental neuroscientists on a systematic quest for the brain's central or "master" processing unit in some localized fragment that integrates simpler component brain elements.[75] Relevant research methods most often involve studying the behavioral effects of focal brain damage or "lesions."[76] Investigators try to dismantle the cranial black box's internal hardware in order to look at the functions of its parts. Pieces of brain play the role of building blocks, which by inference from experiments are presumed to fit together in particular ways that produce the psyche.

The progenitors of modern functional "localizers" first appeared during the nineteenth century. At that time, early investigators began to observe the coarse behavioral effects of crude local brain manipulations. Edward Hitzig and Gustav Fritsch applied electrical current to the right side of a dog's brain and produced involuntary left leg twitches. Paul Broca, working with humans, was able to relate left-sided brain damage to language problems.[77,78]

In this century, experiments in animals produced many behavioral effects of brain damage that pertain also to humans. It was possible, for example, to create inappropriate rage, apathy, bizarre sexuality, and other abnormal states in monkeys and cats by cutting out or electrically stimulating parts of their brains.[79–82]

In the 1940s, electrical probing of the human cortex during

surgery by Wilder Penfield enhanced the detail of maps connecting neuroanatomical addresses with movements of specific body parts.[83] Meanwhile, clinical neurologists and neuropsychologists like Norman Geschwind of the Harvard Medical School[84] and Alexander Luria of Moscow University expanded the scope of lesion studies. Geschwind and his co-workers confirmed earlier reports regarding the function of anatomic structures surrounding the brain's lateral fissure, and their autopsy data were soon followed by corroborating X-ray evidence.[85]

Roger Sperry initiated "split brain" studies in the 1950s by cutting fibers linking the left and right halves of cat brains in order to document asymmetries in resulting behaviors. Epilepsy surgery in the 1960s extended the work to humans and confirmed that speech functions are located in the left side of the brain while contrasting spatial abilities lie on the right. Later, less invasive investigations isolated brain regions nonsurgically, using such functional tools as divided visual fields and "dichotic" listening techniques.[86] These approaches provided the opportunity to create behavioral dissociations despite structurally intact links between the left and right halves of the brain.[87]

In recent years, standardized, quantifiable tasks have come to dominate modular neurobehavioral testing. Neuropsychologists have developed such tools as the Halstead–Reitan Battery, Wisconsin Card Sort, Boston Diagnostic Aphasia Examination, Raven Progressive Matrices, Mini Mental State, Wechsler Memory Scale, and Rey–Osterreith Complex Figure Test.[88,89] CT, MRI, PET, and SPECT scanning machines have also given scientists a profusion of anatomical data through increasingly fine, computer-enhanced resolution of brain images.[90,91]

These approaches have borne a limited amount of fruit, to the extent that a few unexpected experimental results have been obtained. For example, common sense had falsely lured some people into a belief that related behaviors arise in adjacent brain structures. Defects in stroke patients subverted this notion: Problems with muscle control appeared after injury of disparate sites in the forebrain and hindbrain. Aspects of vision and limb sensation showed similar splits in command centers. An inverse principle also became clear: Some abilities that seemed completely unrelated turned out to require the integrity of common brain structures. Examples included the internal sense of body image and expression of emotion, which were both affected by right-sided cerebral damage.[92]

Nevertheless, the central neural command center itself has proved impossible to locate empirically. Most complex properties of the normal intellect, including long-term memory, intelligence, and especially overall "central" processing, do not fit well today into particular anatomic slots.[93] As one eloquent observer[94] has put it, we cannot "either in a specific neurone or brain juice find a precise locus to satisfy our convictions of an operative 'I.'" For investigators in the field, the "hunt" for the human brain's command module never seems to produce a "capture."

The apparent futility of searching for the mind's master control module is a hint that functionalism might not provide the most solid possible grounding for neuropsychiatric assumptions. Psychology and psychiatry must deal with this issue if they are to buttress themselves more securely.

6

Networks

The mind–machine analogy requiring a master control unit likens mental processes to a TV camera. Just as a video monitor scans its environment one patch at a time in sweeps, "serial" computers handle their own operations in linear succession.[1] A control module in the form of a central processing unit must oversee this process from the top down, like a foreman running an assembly line.[2]

This kind of computer design has been able to imitate specific, mechanical human behaviors.[3] It can solve particular types of mathematical problems, play certain kinds of games, provide "expertise" in narrowly circumscribed areas of interest, and display limited pattern recognition.

But humans can do many things that "top-down" computers cannot. Humans more easily compensate for mistakes, fill in missing pieces of the environment, and recognize visual patterns. Top-down automatons lack human judgment, flexibility, common sense, and an ability to infer the unknown. When facing tasks that depart from a stereotype, they must be guided by humans. Like an automobile, each of these machines needs a programmer sitting in the driver's seat.

Much empirical data about human neural "systems" has frustrated top-down modelers of the mind. It has become clear that the feedback and feed-forward control schemes of top-down computing by themselves cannot possibly run the brain. Chemical transmitter bottlenecks, sluggish neuronal components, and nondigital variants of synaptic connections are too slow and inexact to support top-down, cybernetically regulated mental processes. Moreover, noise permeates the brain, and redundant storage wastes such large amounts of memory that even a thousand-billion-billion-fold increase in capacity could not provide adequate compensatory computing power. Yet humans can sort out input from biological sensors like the eye, ear, skin, tongue, and nose in a much finer way than we have a right to expect.[4–10]

Such facts suggest that the brain is not really a serial computer at all. In fact, the brain seems to process data in ways quite different from the wholesale sequential memory searches used by top-down systems.[11] Unlike serial computers, no one unit in the brain encodes particular bits of data, which instead spread as patterns of activity throughout large neuronal populations.[12] In other words, brain coding seems to depend not on individual neural events, but on their statistical properties.[13–17] The mind hence seems able to work with less precise information than is needed by a serial device based on discrete input–output functions.[18–20]

This helps the brain function better than top-down computers in the face of internal structural damage.[21] Unlike top-down computing components, with their sequential flow of program executions, different regions of the brain connect to each other through highly complex reciprocal links.[22,23] These links render the system interactive, with partial damage thus unleashing, through remaining intact structures, compensatory functions not obvious when the whole "system" operates normally. As a result, brain function declines "gracefully" with increasing damage, in contrast to the sudden and catastrophic impact of control-unit breakdown in a serial computer.[24,25]

ᢌ   ᢌ   ᢌ

In order to tackle discrepancies between "top-down," serial computers and the human brain, a new computing analogy has become popular among psychologists in recent years. This "bottom-up" approach has moved the research focus from a postulated master control unit, on "top" of the neural hierarchy and involving gross patterns that are poorly understood,[26] to the microscopic units of brain activity at the "bottom." Investigators thus avoid speculating about the overall command structure of the mind and instead observe directly how individual microunits of the brain interconnect and modify their links with each other.[27] The "bottom-up" approach hence diffuses central control into a probabilistic entity, trading the master module for a more flexible kind of brain organization.

Warren McCulloch (1899–1969) first flirted with this idea in his "principle of redundancy of central command." McCulloch, born in Orange, New Jersey, attended Yale and Columbia, where he earned his medical degree in 1923. He served as an intern at Bellevue Hospital, worked as an instructor in physiological psychology, and then joined a New Haven laboratory investigating the brain of the chimpanzee. At the University of Illinois in 1941, McCulloch, along with Walter Pitts, produced two of the basic papers that have shaped brain science, "A Logical Calculus of the Ideas Immanent in Nervous Activity" and "How We Know Universals: The Perception of Visual and Auditory Forms." In 1952, McCulloch moved to MIT, where he led a team formulating mathematical models of neural networks at the Research Laboratory of Electronics. The products of his collaborative labors included insights into the neurophysiology of vision, the design of reliable neural networks from unreliable elements, and "triadic" logic.[28]

McCulloch's concept of central command redundancy postulates shifts of behavioral control in the brain from one region to another on demand by the environment. His model adapts fixed "neural nets," laid out to process specific types of data under the control of rigid guidelines, to the varied needs of learning theory in the more flexible form of local associative systems.[29-31] Such ideas have helped to create the modern concept of parallel distributive networks in the brain. As Professor Phillip Johnson-Laird, author of *The Computer and the Mind*, describes them, these networks wire

> parallel . . . processors—finite state devices—. . . to each other so as to allow for communication. . . . They . . . pass information to one another. There is no central clock that synchronizes them: each processor springs to life as soon as it receives an adequate input.[32]

Gross anatomical evidence to support this kind of model in neurophysiology first appeared in the early nineteenth century with Pierre Flourens's experiments on pigeons. His results strongly suggested that brain structures house their higher mental functions in no specific locations, but instead diffuse them throughout the cortex.[33-35] Views stemming from Flourens's conclusions remained popular until the 1860s,[36] waned, and revived in the early twentieth century with the work of Karl Lashley (1890–1958).

Lashley attended Johns Hopkins University, worked under the behaviorist Watson, and also collaborated with Shepherd Ivery Franz, a pioneer in studying brain mechanisms of animal intelligence. Later Lashley took the lead in looking at the effect of brain damage on learning in rats and monkeys. His most important work, which showed the limits of localization hypotheses for higher mental functions, was summarized in his 1930 monograph, *Brain Mechanisms and Intelligence*.[37] He reported finding that impairment of memory in animals depends more on the amount than on the site of brain injury. This led him to affirm that control of the most general and abstract mental operations is not easily localized. Instead, the tissue that supports higher intellectual life is "equipotential" no matter where it lies within the brain. Lashley called this last idea the "law of mass action."[38]

Lashley trained other important neuroscientists such as Stanford University's Karl Pribram.[39] In the distributive spirit, Pribram proposed that human memory works like a hologram. Photographs taken by holography differ from ordinary pictures. Every location within a holographic record stores information about each point of an imaged object. Removing pieces of film containing a holographic image therefore does not fully delete any one part of the coded picture; the whole pattern just becomes grainier. Holograms hence provide analogies for possible neural networks and their tendency to spread information from each input throughout many coordinated parallel memory elements, rather than clumping specific data together at one address.[40-44]

Recent laboratory findings, based on neuroimaging techniques like PET, SPECT, CAT, MRI, and evoked electrical potentials in humans as well as single-probe recording in animals, have made it clear that some probabilistic smearing of conscious "control" throughout the brain indeed occurs. The implication at a microscopic level is that functional brain cell types overlap. Each cell can play "multiple roles."[45] This versatility enables the so-called mind modules of the brain to blend each other's information into a common pool.

Vernon Mountcastle of Johns Hopkins[46] discovered supporting evidence for such brain cell relations in a repeating lattice of connections among neuronal units. He showed how these cells, arranged in mutually parallel columns that all run perpendicular to the brain's surface, influence each other's activity.[47-49] Mountcastle's original work centered only on brain sites subserving body sensation. Several years later, however, two other investigators, David Hubel[50] and Torsten Wiesel,[51] obtained equally impressive results from regions of the cortex related to vision.[52] Other research showed columnar links among cells necessary for thinking and planning. A different kind of parallel pattern emerged in a sausagelike brain structure crucial for learning. Its cellular units proved to be stacked in cross-sectional layers. The activity of different cell types in each layer seemed to depend on connections to other cells. Bursts of cellular activity correlated with memory and dream states.[53]

Neurobiology today sees many of these brain architectures as parallel systems with tiers of input–output devices that "extract features" from signals initially provided by sensory channels. A detector organ first registers input and dismantles it into pieces. Each chunk of the input then moves along its own bundle of nerve fibers, through synaptic connections in the brain's "relay" stations, and on to other areas for further analysis. The pieces transmitted at any one time all travel along diffusely distributed parallel circuits simultaneously. Only at the end of the line do the fragments reassemble into the brain's interpreted reconstruction of the world.[54]

Attempts to model all the parallel distributive features of the brain in machines have coalesced during the last decade into the school of thought known as connectionism. This new approach provides computational concepts of the brain as rigorous as the top-down framework, but also seems to bypass some of the serial computer's limitations.[55]

The various connectionist submodels, each adapted to different research goals, all share common properties. They all consist of many simple units. Each unit is analogous to a brain cell or small assembly of cells. The activity of each unit influences and is influenced by others through links of variable strength and either positive or negative valence. Connections hence mimic excitatory and inhibitory synapses, whose converging influences on a particular unit sum to determine the influenced unit's state at any one time. Information in the total network appears as a distributed pattern of activity throughout many units and is processed by the spread of activity. All knowledge retained by the network resides in the total pattern of interunit connection strengths and valences.[56] This knowledge may be graded in the degree of its completeness like a hologram.

As we might expect, many aspects of actual neuropsychological function lend themselves to modeling by artificial connectionist networks. Learning is represented by changes in the strengths of ties between units. Associative features of memory stem from inclusion of the so-called Hebb rule, which says that if two units assume approximately matching states of activity, the link between them will tighten in the appropriate direction of valence. Because of this, networks "seeded" by partial memory fragments will tend to spill into a total pattern analogous to the entire memory. Under normal circumstances, the chain of states leading from one memory pattern to the next proceeds relatively smoothly, modeling our commonly experienced stream of consciousness.[57–60]

Supervening rules may be imposed on summed, converging influences at a particular unit to influence that unit's state. Changing such rules diffusely throughout an entire network will thereby produce global "modulation." The maneuver will change the overall state of processing without producing a discrete input–output signal of its own at any particular locality, as would happen in a serial processing system.[61,62]

Changing a rule simulates the diffuse actions of chemical neuromodulators in the brain. These substances fall somewhere between classic synaptic transmitters and hormones. Acetylcholine, serotonin, norepinephrine, and dopamine, some of which serve as classical transmitters, also function as neuromodulators. In this capacity, they are produced by small cell body groups at the brain's core. Radial fiber projections from these sites allow the substances access to widespread and diverse target regions within the central nervous system. The core cell groups send their signals outward at a more leisurely pace than focal transmitting agents and have relatively longer-lasting impact. As a result, though specific sensory signals cannot travel along modulatory pathways, neuromodulators appear to many neuroscientists as the ideal substrates for overall regulation of conscious states, including wakefulness, various stages of sleep, and dreaming.[63–65]

Modulators like dopamine, norepinephrine, and serotonin all increase the so-called signal-to-noise ratio of target brain cell behavior profiles. These substances exaggerate unit output responses to excitatory input, but in complementary fashion also intensify the effects of inhibitory input; hence, such modulators sharpen the input–output properties of target neurons in toto. They have the same effect on the overall signal-to-noise ratio of a subject's gross behavior during experimental stimulus-detection tasks. Stimulant drugs like amphetamines, which exert their effects through neuromodulating intermediaries, boost the ability of humans to discriminate selected events from extraneous phenomena. That is, amphetamines reduce both the number of undetected test stimuli and the frequency of false alarms. Modulators like dopamine, norepinephrine, and serotonin thereby sharpen the input–output properties not only of target neurons but of overall behavior as well.[66,67]

The neuropsychiatric hypothesis that defective modulators cause mental abnormalities has found its way into neural network theory. Concepts of modulatory failure have appeared regarding depression, mania, anxiety disorders, and attention-deficit syndromes.[68] A specific disturbance in the continuity of successive stable memory states has been advanced to model the so-called "dissociative" psychiatric disorders.[69] Inherited mental illnesses and those acquired early in life have been blamed on links between parallel brain channels weakened by synaptic problems during infancy.[70–72]

Simulated psychotic behavior in artificial parallel processing systems seems to suggest a noise-enhancing role for dopamine in schizophrenia.[73–75] Moreover, researchers are finding that simulations of frontal lobe "pruning" imbue parallel networks with schizophrenic-like behavior. Pruning spontaneously pares away less frequently utilized synaptic connections during the course of normal development. Biological pruning has been simulated in artificial parallel networks through a rule expunging weaker links between processing units over time. Such outcomes generate models for the pathogenic role of pruning during the most common age of onset for schizophrenia.[76]

Pruning in parallel circuits constitutes an analogy to the ideas of Charles Darwin. It reprises the Darwinian mechanism by which competition weeds out less "fit" organisms in the natural world. Some theorists, adapting this concept to brain components, have postulated that a myriad of unconscious processes, subserved by parallel brain channels, compete for access to the final selective pathway into consciousness. Neural network modulation could well be recast to represent the natural background for such a phenomenon. Cortical arousal by the brain's core might mediate selective resonance of one among many specific modulatory options jockeying to take over the diffuse workings of the whole brain.[77]

In such a competitive system, steep gain increases in response to stimulus input, combined with the Hebb rule and chemical arousal, could create explosive bursts of neural activity and hence discontinuous jumps between discrete aggregate states of neuronal networks. Researchers have found evidence of such structured complexity within brain systems supporting visual abilities and the sense of smell. In the words of one expert, they have identified a tendency for "vast collections of neurons to shift abruptly and simultaneously from one complex activity pattern to another in response to the smallest of inputs." Graphic "phase portraits" of simulated systems have also exhibited such behavior. Their patterns reveal the different states between which virtual competing neuronal systems explosively leap back and forth. Such phenomena represent a mathematical property called "chaos."[78–82]

The idea of neural chaos can be understood by comparing it to its antithesis. Neural non-chaos is typified by deterministic features of learning in primitive organisms. Simple animals usually have nervous systems much less complex than the human brain. Their neurons are large in size and few in number, and hence can be easily seen under a microscope by researchers. Each individual cell always appears in the same place with respect to other cells; its location does not vary from animal to animal. Junction sites between such cells tend to be predictable.[83]

These very properties have kept the technical challenges of research with simple animals manageable, but they also make such nervous systems inappropriate for comparison to more advanced neural networks relevant to human behavior. The brains of intelligent organisms like man, quite different from those of primitive organisms, consist of small, numerous neurons whose locations and connections vary from individual to individual even within one species. The orderliness that a determinist can hope to see in the interneuronal signals of simple animals breaks down in organisms closer to our own human form. In these higher vertebrates, even the regularity of columnar brain cell lattices is puny compared to surrounding seas of neural noise.[84] Many relevant brain regions interact not only through organized nerve fiber bundles, but also through disorderly links that complicate any research program bent on reducing human consciousness to a neat architecture. It is strikingly true that those "reticular" structures which lie at the brain's center and are vital for maintaining consciousness are most dominated by disorder.

In the context of these observations, chaos theory seems more appropriate than does orderly determinism. In fact, chaos seems to some as though it might be the very attribute that creates mental flexibility. Chaotic features thus help to make neural network theory a popular current alternative to failed serial computing theories of the mind.[85]

ફ   ફ   ફ

All these considerations notwithstanding, there are problems with the connectionistic view of mind and brain. First, gross parallel network performance differs from human behavior in that artificial systems learn mainly from errors and require a teacher, while a human can learn by himself and often exploits his own successes. Second, idealized parallel networks on a microscopic level do not completely correspond to any actual type of neural system.[86] Third, as Johnson-Laird has stated,

> whatever form parallel processing takes, it cannot compute anything that could not be computed by a single serial processor. . . . Nor can it make intractable search problems tractable: they are to computation what Malthus's doctrine of population growth is to civilization. What parallel processing can do is speed up tractable

procedures, to allow several processors to carry out the same task so that it is less affected by noise or damage to the system. . . .[87]

Some researchers addressing objections to connectionism have come up with an alternative. They have proposed that if standard parallel computing architecture cannot model all the workings of the mind, perhaps quantum-mechanical analogues will fill the bill.

General characteristics of "quantum computing" have been worked out in the abstract. A quantum computer has all the capabilities of standard parallel computers, but it can also represent complicated "superpositions" of many standard computational states. Because of this ability, as one commentator explains, "a quantum computer is capable of a kind of quantum parallelism which, unlike conventional parallel processing, is not restricted as regards the number of tasks that can be performed simultaneously."[88] Therefore, a problem whose solution is only probable or possible with a standard computational technique may be soluble with certainty in the quantum mode.[89]

However, no quantum computer has ever actually been built. Hence, in the absence of any real test device that might run simulations of the human psyche, judgments about quantum computing must rest on abstract argument alone. Since the quantum approach reduces data to integers,[90] we might suspect that it retains the numerical myopia of all computational approaches to psychology. Indeed, quantum computing as the ultimate functionalistic metaphor for mind may be the most numerically self-referent model of all.

Neither quantum analogues, chaos theory, Darwinian metaphors, modulatory mechanisms, nor other parallel distributive concepts provide totally satisfying solutions to the problems posed by standard serial-computing metaphors for the mind. The question that we must now ask is whether any complete answers are possible.

7

The Downside of Machine Metaphors

*I*s it meaningful to ask how many subunits, circuits, and cross-connections among channels[1] will turn a computer into a mind? Is it possible to measure how complicated computing machines need to be in order to attain consciousness?

These issues, since they are quantitative, involve numbers. Moreover, because computer operations themselves can be encoded in numerical terms,[2] the pertinent quantities are self-referent.

Self-reference of any sort, including numerical or computational self-reference, generates paradoxes. Paradoxical statements refer in a circular way back to their own truth or falsehood.[3]

There are many known examples of paradoxes. Epimenides of Crete paradoxically asserted that "all Cretans are liars." Bertrand Russell conjured up the conundrum of the "barber who shaves those in his town who do not shave themselves." Groucho Marx said that he would not join any club that would accept him as a member. All such expressions are really variations on the prototypical paradox, "this sentence is false."[4,5]

This last, core assertion illustrates how self-referent paradoxes grow from ambiguities of scale with respect to the measurement of truth. The truth of the statement "this sentence is false" cannot be pinned down because if the entire sentence considered as a whole from the outside is true, then its internal sense applies, rendering it false. On the other hand, if the entire sentence is false, then the internal assertion of falsity itself becomes false, rendering the entire sentence true. The truth-reference of the paradox thus shuttles between part and whole without ever settling down.[6]

Bertrand Russell attempted in his ramified theory of "types" to construct abstractive hierarchies aimed at bypassing such paradoxical tangles of part and whole. Russell ranked sentences about the truth of other sentences in categories according to their degree of abstraction. With increasing rank, Russell's superordinate sentence "types" subsumed more and more numerous subtypes of lower rank. Hence, the theory of types became a structure shot through with self-similar levels of hierarchical scale. This arrangement seemed to account for the blurred distinctions between part and whole characteristic of paradox.[7,8]

But Russell's effort ultimately failed. Self-referent paradoxes and their infinite regressions of logic continued to arise. The quest for scale-invariant, universally nonparadoxical statements ran amok and became an endless hierarchy of repeating self-similarities without a ceiling. Relativized, self-contradictory dichotomies of part versus whole never stopped bouncing pointlessly across the boundaries of scale.

Self-referent paradoxes in fact may occur with or without hierarchies of type. They appear whenever confusion arises between the phrase "there exists" and the expression "for all."[9] These two complementary pairs of words can change a statement such as "a dog has four legs" into others like "at least one dog exists with four legs" or "all dogs have four legs." They are the so-called "quantifiers"[10] of formal logic.

The universal quantifier "for all" sets up the potential for paradox whenever a predicate referring to "all" members of a set is itself also considered as a possible member of the set. The most famous example of a self-contradiction resulting from such a situation is Russell's "class of all classes not belonging to themselves."[11,12]

The existential quantifier "there exists" helps in cementing self-referent paradoxes insofar as its own logical reciprocity[13] with the universal quantifier becomes blurred. Normally the elemental domain of existence does not encroach on universal realms. The statement "at least one dog exists with four legs" remains distinct from the sentence "all dogs have four legs." When existence is confused with universality, however, different levels of discourse are conflated. This paradoxically places parts of sets in one-to-one correspondence with their respective wholes.

The mathematicians Kurt Gödel (1906–1978) and Alan Turing (1912–1954) explicitly related insights about self-reference, quantifiers, numerical scale, and paradoxes to computing theory. Several other thinkers, including Alfred Tarski[14] and Alonzo Church, also made important contributions.

Gödel was born in what later became Czechoslovakia, attended the University of Vienna, and earned his doctorate as a logician in 1930. One year later he published his most famous of many important papers, proving that arithmetic is logically incomplete. In 1938 and 1939, Gödel gave a series of lectures that laid the groundwork for a radically new theory of mathematical sets. He moved to the United States and worked at the Institute for Advanced Studies in Princeton from 1940 until he retired.[15]

Turing was born in London and attended Cambridge. In 1937, his paper "On Computable Numbers with an Application to the Entscheidungsproblem" demarcated limits on computability by showing the unpredictability of mechanical "halting" behavior. His concepts of computing also broke German codes for the British military during World War II. Turing's article of 1950, "Computing Machinery and Intelligence," laid out many powerful concepts for use in future research. However, he died, possibly by his own hand, while still in his prime.[16,17]

Turing and Gödel both addressed the issues of self-reference, quantifiers, numerical scale, and paradoxes in novel ways. Gödel did so by constructing formal statements about arithmetical computation. These statements themselves employed an arithmetically coded and therefore self-referent language. Gödel used the self-referently numbered encodement of his propositions to prove that arithmetic as a whole, in its axiomatic form, contains insoluble quandaries.[18-20] Turing related such quandaries to the concrete behavior of computing machines.

Conclusions akin to those deduced by Gödel and Turing not only discredited the entire formalist program for arithmetic and numerical computation, they undercut programs enthroning empirical measurement as well. These also buckled under the weight of internal quantitative self-contradictions.[21-28]

As Kant and Berkeley pointed out, we have no purely logical grounds on which to assume that measurable or computable quantities like space, time, and mass are the real stuff of the world. These concepts instead come from distortions inherent in the artifice of self-referent numbers. Man-made ideas alone create the measurable quantities and mechanistic biases of traditional physics.[29-33]

Mathematically oriented philosophers have said much that pertains to this problem. However, quantitative self-contradictions go uncontested in modern nonmathematical thought because people outside mathematics, even if otherwise well-informed, generally overlook the theoretical assumptions behind numerically based practices in our society.[34]

The philosopher Herbert Marcuse, espousing the "Frankfurt School" of social criticism discussed in Chapter 10 of this book, has amplified this point. Marcuse wrote that number-worshiping mind-sets cannot even recognize their own conceptual myopia within our technically oriented culture; instead, they degenerate into the "false consciousness" of a self-perpetuating closed system. The very efficiency of applied quantitative technology in achieving self-justifying ends winds up predetermining experience "*a priori*." Hence, modern technological man, including the quantitative psychologist, dooms himself to believe that precise quantification of nature can reveal "absolute truth," while in reality measurement remains "a specific method and technique" with self-deceptive, self-perpetuating flaws.[35]

Resulting distortions make the world appear as a well-oiled

"system" with internal numerical relations in total command; defects in the system appear as mere glitches easily fixed by technology alone. Reality shrinks to a mass of empirical data poised for number crunching in science's quest for the ultimate equation, while overexpansive computing metaphors destroy the possibility of a coherent epistemology by crumpling it into self-referent paradox. Such a warped outlook locks people with self-referently numerical biases into futile cycles of tail-chasing, constantly seeking new quantitative routes out of complications born from number worship itself. The quantitative mind set of our technological culture hence actively obliterates any chance to break out of its own limited perspective.[36,37]

Human beings cannot trust the fallout from their theories about the world if they ignore the sources of their own thinking processes. The reason is that, as one perceptive observer has noted, "there is philosophy implicit in everything we do, although it remains, for the most part, outside of our awareness."[38] This is true even for specifically quantitative fields of scientific inquiry.

The eminent historian of science Thomas Kuhn has argued that the assumptions and biases of a scientific discipline prejudice not only its theories but also the very kinds of experiments and data that it deems proper.[39] Kuhn is well-qualified to make such a case. He earned his degree as a physicist at Harvard under J. B. Conant and, after teaching a course on the philosophical and historical underpinnings of science, proceeded to explore the subject in masterful depth. His important book *The Structure of Scientific Revolutions* shows that science is an evolving chain of viewpoints, each conditioned by its historical predecessors and imposing its own paradigmatic slant.[40–42] Quantitative biases surely number among such slants.

The assertions of science not only describe matters of physical fact, but also phrase them in ways that include those actions by which a scientist biases experimental measurements. This is because equations often assume an active form, incorporating either implicitly or explicitly the way in which an experimental manipulation brings about a physical change of state. For example, expressions describing the solid, liquid, and gaseous phases of water imply the experimenter's actions in changing the temperature of an aqueous system. This aspect of science illustrates that even empirical measurement depends on the activity of scientists as subjective agents, since a mistaken design in their manipulations, producing misleading laboratory data, can invade and sully an entire theoretical structure.[43,44]

Modern physics recognizes this fact. Mind and self have entered the realm of the late-twentieth-century physicist as he shifts his gaze from the illusion of objective events toward the subjectivity of quantum-mechanical observations and relativistic reference frames.[45] An "anthropic" version of physics even suggests that the presence of living minds in our universe affects the form of quantum laws.[46] The origin of "hard" physical science in the biases of the psyche thus doubles back on itself, and many physicists are now working to address the consequences.

Just as early-twentieth-century scientists could not fit the quantum world of the atom into an outmoded nineteenth-century material framework independent of mind, psychiatrists who try to force the general methods of quantitative science on psychology today are headed toward the wrong goal.[47] Early research into the abstruse realm of electrons, protons, and neutrons showed that the theories of Newton were only approximations of general physical law in the special case of everyday phenomena. In the same spirit, but at a metalevel beyond, the self-reference of psychology reveals that the computability of quantitative science itself is only a special case of some larger mode by which humans understand the world.

Quantitative psychology, even more than other areas of scientific inquiry, must deal with the issues of self-reference. The active self-reference of a scientist's experimental controls should serve as a model for the more general dependence of all ideas on prejudices molding every creative thought process. If the content of science includes experiments, then the content of thought must subsume its own development. The whole of mental function contains more than the sum of its parts, since it must also include the means by which mind chooses to shape itself in free acts of continual autoinvention.

Human progress in all its guises requires creative confrontation with the self, and that need becomes most acute in the study of mind. The challenge cannot be met mechanically, since active choices by the psychologist must themselves constantly be checked. The student of mind must direct his scrutiny not only at experimental data but also at the personal wellsprings of his own hypotheses. Psychologists and psychiatrists must engage in "thinking about thinking," which requires an interplay of factors that is beyond computing machines or the rigid paradigms of technical, applied, quantitative science. It is for this reason that quantitative rigor will forever elude psychology. As the mathematician and philosopher of science Jacob Bronowski has put it:

> There is an essential difficulty in casting . . . [psychologically oriented] disciplines into an axiomatic system. They are limited, more severely and more consistently than the natural sciences, by the self-reference that underlies them everywhere. . . . The axiomatic method as such may be unworkable in these studies, and whatever . . . is discovered for them in the future will (I think) not be of this traditional kind.[48]

Hence, attempts like those of the behaviorist Clark Hull to create a purely axiomatic superstructure for psychology akin to arithmetical formalism[49,50] must fail. As Bronowski wrote, "the knowledge of the self cannot be formalized because it cannot be closed, even provisionally."[51] The open self-reference of positivistic biases as psychological phenomena themselves blocks the hunger of positivistic psychology for final self-knowledge. Self-contradictions exist in modern psychology and psychiatry largely because their technical biases ignore this fact.

Despite their quantitative bent and unlike subsequent researchers, early experimental psychologists of the nineteenth century recognized such limits. They saw clearly that they could not shrivel mind into precisely measurable processes without doing violence to self-understanding. Fechner applied statistics to psychology merely because of an imperfect match between subjective experience and objectively measurable phenomena. Helmholtz understood that linear scientific measurement pertains only in a very limited way to "interwoven" elements of the psyche. Even Wundt believed that mental processes transcend measurable mechanisms and involve active participation by the mental agent in ordering perceptions. Rather than extending exact measurement beyond "directly accessible . . . organs of sense of movement," Wundt relegated higher and more complex mental domains to qualitative study. He looked at them through the lenses of historical, cultural, and religious scholarship, which he grouped under the category of *Völkerpsychologie*. Pioneers like Fechner, Helmholtz, and Wundt all understood that the self will remain forever beyond our grasp if it is sought only in a numerical form.[52]

However, successors have become blind to the bootstraps by which they suspend the foundations of their own quantitative research methods.[53] Systematic exclusion of introspective self-reflection from the psychiatric lexicon in recent years has distorted the thrust of new facts amassed by researchers. The very controls built into experiments have slanted the viewpoints of investigators and the behavior of research subjects against subjective self-reflection. Experimental design itself has thus guaranteed empirical support for the idea of a measurable and neatly parceled "physiology" of consciousness.

The paradigm of "lesion" studies has fractured mental function into an artificially ordered ensemble of mechanistic "modules." "Split brain" experimental research in particular has locked the brain into modules by isolating regions of the cortex, either functionally or anatomically, as a precondition of tests for behavioral changes. Moreover, split brain techniques, in trying to keep subjects active enough to behave in an alert manner, have employed methods that spare arousal functions in the brainstem. The resulting experiments thus skirt the whole issue of chaotic non-modularity at the reticulated core of the brain.

In complementary fashion, during many investigations, drugs that keep animal subjects tractable have affected behavioral outcomes by suppressing either consciousness or free movement. Reliance on "controlled" research interventions like anesthesia, drug-induced paralysis, and mechanical restraints can distort behavioral outcomes as potently as brain lesions.[54–56]

Stepwise mechanical styles of thought[57] bias research designs toward computational approaches to the psyche that are fraught with internal self-contradictions. The issue of "dishabituation" is a prime example. Animals often lose interest in stimuli that are repeated monotonously at predictable intervals. The intensity of their responses may decrease and the responses may ultimately disappear during the process called habituation. However, change in the stimulus may induce a sudden return or even an overshoot in response. Several investigators have suggested mechanisms for this dishabituative increase,[58,59] but as a general program in the brain it seems paradoxical. Any participating system of neurons would have to keep tuned to stimulus features based on information that is by definition not yet known. No general program can be designed to carry out this task.[60]

Phenomena like dishabituation illustrate how psychology's mechanical research methods, designed precisely to exclude all opportunity for qualitative self-understanding, doom themselves to defeat. Advocates of empirical psychology, by presuming that our minds can be known to us only through quantitation of behavior, thus degrade our picture of the self. Scholars are encouraged to venerate their own arithmetical creations in a kind of circular autoidolatry.

Medically oriented clinical psychiatrists are far from immune to this sort of trap. The standard Western medical approach to illness today assumes that the body functions as a machine, illness results from mechanical breakage, and the doctor acts as a repairman. The result is inadequate attention to the intangible factors operating in these infirmities. Symptoms are merely categorized in a disease taxonomy, and their relation to the entire life history of the patient is fragmented and obscured.[61]

To the extent that psychiatrists look more and more on the mechanical aspects of their work as a grandiose scientific sacrament that totally commands their actions, both research and clinical practice threaten to devour themselves in self-defeating quantitation. Thus, as self-referent numbers emerge as a universal pseudostandard of explanation, everyone may be crunched into numbers.

           za.   za.   za.

"Intentionality" is the crucial concept not encompassed by quantitative psychology, with its penchant for empirical measurement and computer metaphors.

Daniel Dennett, head of the Center for Cognitive Studies at Tufts University,[62,63] and John Haugeland, professor of philosophy at the University of Pittsburgh,[64] point out that the central idea behind intentionality is "aboutness." Intentional phenomena refer to something outside themselves.[65] Through contextual[66] links, an intentional entity can feed and grow, transcending its own boundaries and spilling beyond itself into what it is not.

Intentionality in this academic sense is not exactly synonymous with its common meaning of aim or purpose.[67,68] Rigorous usage of the term intentionality retains these everyday associations but also subsumes other words such as hope, belief, and imagination[69,70]; hoping, believing, and imagining are all intentional mental acts.[71] They meet the definition of intentionality because they refer to objects outside themselves. Owen Flanagan, chairman of the philosophy department at Duke University, shows this nicely in his book *The Science of the Mind* by pointing out that when "people desire that _____ , hope that_____ , expect that _____, perceive that _____, and so on, . . . whatever [object] fills in the blank is the intentional content of the mental act."[72]

John Searle, Mills Professor of the Philosophy of Mind and Language at the University of California at Berkeley, has distinguished between intentional meaning and the formal structure of nonintentional sentences.[73] Flanagan illustrates the point by showing how sentences with intentional verbs are distinct from and transcend rules that bind nonintentional sentences. For example, he writes that

> whereas it follows from "The president is a Republican" and "Bush is the president" that "Bush is a Republican," it does not follow from "John believes that the president is a Republican" and "Bush is the president" that "John believes that Bush is a Republican." John, after all, might not know that Bush is the president.

Flanagan explains that in the above exercise, replacing one noun with an "identical" term does not maintain the truth or falsity of sentences with intentional verbs in the same way that it maintains the status of sentences with nonintentional verbs.[74]

The rebellious thinker Franz Brentano (1838–1917) first forged a clear link between intentionality and subjective mind. Brentano, ordained as a Roman Catholic priest in 1864, taught philosophy at Würzburg until, rejecting the Pope's infallibility and marrying at the age of 42, he left his professorial post. Brentano continued teaching and working in Vienna until retiring in 1893.[75–77] He wrote that "every mental phenomenon is characterized by what the Scholastics of the Middle Ages called . . . intentional . . . reference. . . ."[78] This doctrine, now known as "Brentano's Thesis," implies that any form of psychology adequate to deal with subjectivity requires a vocabulary that includes intentional terms.[79]

Searle has restated Brentano's requirement in modern idiom by asserting that "minds have mental contents; specifically they have semantic contents."[80] Flanagan has also rephrased Brentano's Thesis in contemporary terms by suggesting that "minds display "an 'aboutness' that tables and chairs lack."[81] He remarks that even "books are only derivatively about something: Anna Karenina is about Anna Karenina only because we attach meaning to ink marks on paper."[82]

Such views hold that the mind works by intentionally directing itself toward objects of mental contents through a contextual reach beyond the constraints of formal, merely "syntactical" structure.[83] Moreover, the mind not only operates by way of intentionality; its very nature[84,85] is intentional. William Barrett, former head of New York University's philosophy department, has explained this perspective as follows:

> Consciousness . . . is . . . not a determinate kind of thing at all. . . . If we want to talk about consciousness, we are able only to talk about the objects of which we are conscious. When we try to look into it, we look through it and past it. If I try to examine my "blue mood" of the moment, I find only things in the world that now strike me as "blue." The nature of consciousness is to point beyond itself—to whatever datum it is conscious of.[86]

Hence, as Bronowski has stated, mental processes cannot be merely logical. Instead, "the logic of the mind differs from formal logic in its ability to overcome and indeed exploit the ambivalences of self-reference, so that they become the instruments of [expansive] imagination."[87] Intentionality thereby casts the mind as an entity unbounded by an assignable objective domain.[88–90]

In contrast, the organizing concept of modern computing is a program that manipulates only abstract symbols and is devoid of implicit intentional content. All computer software programs, unlike unpredictable human behavior, can be reduced to a set of well-defined rules and formal mechanisms. Computational software languages hence consist only of syntactical properties without intrinsic meaning.[91–93] As Hearnshaw has emphasized,

> there is no more intentionality in . . . [the purely formal symbolism of a] computer program than there is in the printed pages of a book. . . . True, the computer, unlike the book, is dynamic, it involves processes in time, and is not merely the static record of the results of thought. It can provide answers to problems that the unaided human mind cannot provide. But this does not imply inten-

tionality. A simple calculating machine can give answers
that no human being can immediately give; but no one
has suggested that it "thinks." Nor does a computer
"think" in the full sense of the word even though it . . .
[might] momentarily fool an interlocuter.[94]

Charles Babbage (1792–1871) conceived the abstract, formal,
nonintentional design of our present serial computer technology
in the nineteenth century. Babbage, born in England into a
wealthy banking family and educated at Cambridge, devoted
much of his own money to developing his ideas. In collaboration
with Byron's daughter Ada Lovelace, he invented a workable
blueprint for the first programmable computer, his "difference
engine." The machine, designed before the advent of modern
electronics, was to operate via mechanical gears and levers. Its
construction was never finished, but much of it still exists in the
Science Museum of London. Babbage received enough recognition for his work to win a prestigious academic position in 1823,
when he became Lucasian Professor of Mathematics at Cambridge.[95]

In the 1920s, R. V. L. Hartley made the first attempts at a truly
formal treatment of information theory that might apply to a wide
variety of computing hardwares. Alan Turing in 1936 further
defined general principles for computing machines in universal
terms. Claude Shannon then designed the paradigmatic abstract
circuit design for digital computers according to the formal dic-
tates of Boole's logical algebra. John Von Neumann, about whom
more will be said in Chapter 8, invented the stored "software"
program during the 1940s.

Norbert Wiener (1894–1964) and others completed the formal
theory of information in its mature, fully nonintentional form.
Wiener was born in Cambridge, Massachusetts and rapidly
proved to be a mathematical prodigy, graduating from Tufts University at age 14 and obtaining his doctorate from Harvard at 18.
He became a faculty member at MIT at 25 and went on to break
new ground in many areas of mathematics, especially those con-

nected with electrical engineering. His collaboration with Arturo Rosenblueth at the Harvard Medical School and others spawned cybernetics, the theory of control relationships between man and machine.[96] Wiener's approach to data processing, in parallel with those of Shannon and Weaver, defined information in terms of a numerical measurement independent of source or intentional meaning. Systems accessible to such methods were deemed to have only a known number of possible states and to run according to rigid rules. The relevant equations simply required that in each case for which information is to be measured, a question must be posed and all possible answers enumerated ahead of time. Formalized information thus emerged as the degree of uncertainty in assigning a correct answer.[97]

Reliance on such generalized, symbolic concepts of information has allowed software design in serial computers to accommodate any sort of program whatsoever; the generality of programming lets it apply to a wide variety of machines. However, general programs specify no machine in particular and also denote no intrinsic, unique intentional meaning. This is what drives a wedge of incommensurability between the dead world of computable syntax and subjective meaning within the living mind.[98,99]

Searle's inspired "Chinese Room Argument" illustrates this last point through an analogy. Searle imagined himself as a monolingual English speaker in a room alone. He fantasized that in his possession was a book for translating Chinese into English. The book did not actually contain the means to learn Chinese, but only provided formal rules by which to transform symbols from one language into another. People outside the room slipped him messages to translate. Searle suggested that as he learned the rules and became adept at his task, his performance would approach the efficiency of a computer.[100]

Searle underscored the inability of observers outside the "Chinese Room" to distinguish his rule-following performance from that of a computer. He suggested that his identification with a machine mirrors the way he set up his thought experiment: The meaning of his translations was to be withheld from him. He invoked this provision to show that intentionality is the unique identifying property of subjective mind[101] and thus relegated formal mechanisms to a category altogether different from the human psyche.

Searle also suggested that parallel distributive processing innovations are no more intentional than other computer models of the human mind. He illustrated the intentional poverty of connectionism by extending his Chinese Room argument to that of a "Chinese Gym." Searle's gym was a large room filled with English speakers who understood no Chinese, but each had a rule book for symbol translation. He observed that even without any single speaker understanding Chinese, "the system" could correctly respond to Chinese questions. Searle therefore concluded that "computationally, serial and parallel systems are equivalent. . . . You can't get semantically loaded thought contents from formal computations alone, whether they are done in serial or parallel."[102] Hence, parallel processing does not negate the Chinese Room argument.

Connectionism, like serial computing, is really just another mechanical scheme, albeit one that claims to conjure consciousness as if by magic out of competing parallel subsystems. Connectionists avoid discussion of subjective intentionality on the grounds that conscious introspection may not jibe with the subterranean mode by which multiple parallel unconscious mental processes are supposed to operate.[103] Therefore, instead of intentional issues, parallelists end up concentrating on the same old formal learning paradigms invented by empirical behaviorists.[104–106] Meanwhile, the deepest origins of conscious thought remain unexplained.

Even connectionist analogues in holograms, reconstructed from a sampling of definite data points, lack intrinsic intentionality. And chaotic consequences of parallel systems create abstract "phase spaces" with branching structures whose self-similarities at different scales suggest paradox. These are additional hints that parallel neural networks fail to transcend nonintentional connundra. Syntactical limits that make serial systems inadequate explanations for mental phenomena apply to parallel distributive models as well.[107]

Quantum-mechanical systems and their relevant computational analogues may also lack real intentionality. Subatomic quantum phenomena and their statistical "wave functions" evolve over time in a mechanical way, like a machine, when left undisturbed at a minute scale. Their behavior becomes unpredictable, i.e., their wave functions "collapse," only when an experimental measurement magnifies quantum effects to a size that humans can observe. The implications of this change are a subject of ongoing scientific debate. Some quantum physicists see wave function collapse as evidence that subatomic particles are inherently unruly. Others see the same phenomenon as an unpredictable extrinsic effect of conscious human intervention in the otherwise collectively ordered world of quantum probability laws. Until this controversy resolves itself, the status of quantum computing as a means of transcending limits on machine analogies in psychology must remain in doubt.[108–111]

Hence, the relationship between subjective psychology and the quantitative neurosciences remains a source of difficulty for philosophers to this day. Despite all efforts to establish "bridge laws" between mental and nonintentional domains, the issues generated by Brentano's phenomenology still stand as unmet challenges. A great divide persists today between partisans who embrace intentional concepts and those who prefer more mechanical approaches.[112] Yet, as Flanagan wisely says,

> Thus far we know of only one . . . system that without doubt possesses [intentional] features . . . , namely, Homo sapiens. To be sure, it is possible that . . . other systems may possess these features. . . . Nevertheless, . . . if a brilliant young scientist told me he wanted to spend his career trying to understand intentionality . . . , I would tell him to spend relatively more time looking at creatures that have these features, and relatively less at the . . . systems that might.[113]

8

Meaning in Gauge Fields

*I*f computer metaphors and numbers by themselves fail to account for the peculiar intentionality of the psyche, a question arises: Is it possible to construct a "larger" psychology that is competent to handle intentional meaning without sacrificing numerical precision completely?

The quantitative approach may well prove to be only a limiting case within a more comprehensive kind of mental science. It may yet be possible to retain numbers as one tool among many in a truly constructive, flexible understanding of the mind.[12]

The discipline of metamathematics may provide a means of achieving such a goal. Metamathematics, as the mode of inquiry responsible for bringing arithmetical paradoxes to light, fully encompasses mathematics proper, but speaks beyond it in more general terms. Metamathematical ideas have the potential to produce a mode of inquiry that incorporates numbers and yet also deals effectively with self-reference and intentional meaning.

Novel approaches to psychology might capitalize on the fact that even the most rarefied quantitative ideas of the past have never been purely self-referent; they have always implied physically intentional meanings beyond their own formal structure. Apollonius' work on conic sections gave rise to the physics of Kepler. Descartes' analytic geometry found its way into Copernican astronomy and Galilean mechanics. Newton invented the calculus in order to describe physical movements of real objects in space and on earth. Matrix theory formed a basis for quantum physics. Non-Euclidean geometries permitted Einstein to create his general relativity theory.[3,4]

Psychology may be able to build on this pattern of precedents, generalize them, and thereby supersede dichotomies between quantitative neuroscience and spiritual metaphor. The proper metamathematical leap, transcending mere arithmetic but not rejecting it out of hand, might show how intentional, supra-arithmetical aspects of the psyche are both unquantifiable and yet also real.[5]

Two newer branches of mathematics honed from metamathematical ideas have attributes that can guide us in looking for a better approach to psychology. These are Abraham Robinson's "nonstandard" analysis, which has simplified Newton's approach to the calculus,[6–9] and Paul Cohen's "non-Cantorian" set theory, which has freed infinite numbers from old, intuitively bound biases.[10–14] Both systems of thought extend the horizons of mathematics beyond the standard purview of more traditional approaches. Both deal with issues that transcend formal systems. Both retain the concepts of more orthodox theories as valid though restricted cases within their own larger frameworks. These are all properties that psychology might bear in mind during its search for a metamathematical foundation.

The mathematical giant John Von Neumann predicted that we will need a softening of rigid, formalistic restrictions on number theory in order to relate mind and matter. It is hard to imagine a more authoritative source for this forecast. Von Neumann, born in Budapest in 1903, was already a master of mathematics in childhood. He received his education in Berlin and Zurich and then emigrated to the United States, where he made profound contributions to many important aspects of his field. He served on the Atomic Energy Commission and was a faculty member of the Institute for Advanced Study in Princeton. In 1946 at the Moore School of Electrical Engineering in Philadelphia, Von Neumann headed a group that invented ENIAC, the first digital computer.

He went on to publish work defining the basis for information storage in the next four generations of modern computing devices and elaborated the mathematical basis of game strategies. Shortly before his death in 1957, he advanced new ideas relating probability and error theory to the workings of the central nervous system.[15,16]

Von Neumann wrote that while the brain may well be relevant to mental faculties, "logics and mathematics in the CNS, when viewed as languages, must structurally be essentially different from those languages to which our common experience refers." He hypothesized that "programs" in the brain diverge from all conventional computer software; the challenge lies in mastering them with means beyond mathematics as we now know it. Von Neumann suggested a direction for future research by viewing mathematics as "a secondary language, built on the primary language truly used by the central nervous system." He speculated that the "message system" of mind and brain might be identified by searching for a flexible metacode with "less logical and arithmetical depth than what we normally are used to."[17]

In order to completely reformulate our own perspective on arithmetic in a way that will serve psychology adequately,[18] a specific liberating step, drawing on Von Neumann's ideas, might be needed. To understand this step, we should be open to the possibility of taking psychological investigation beyond mechanism and materialism into the realm of field theory, expanded beyond its present quantitative framework.

Numerically anchored fields have already proven themselves by infusing the physical sciences with great explanatory power. Albert Einstein, the greatest physicist of the twentieth century, acknowledged that the invention of field theory was "the most important event in physics since Newton's time." Einstein said that fields led to "the creation of new concepts" and "a new picture of reality" which proved grander yet more economical than Newton's older ideas because they eliminated any need for "material actors."[19]

Some imaginative psychologists have anticipated the possible relevance of expanded field structures to their discipline. Kurt Lewin (1890–1947), for example, created a field model for use in Gestalt psychology. Lewin, a native of eastern Prussia, studied at the University of Berlin, where he attended the philosophical lectures of Ernst Cassirer and met a group of innovative psychologists at the laboratory of Carl Stumpf. After service in the German army and a battle wound during World War I, Lewin returned to the University of Berlin as a teacher and made contact with the Gestaltists Max Wertheimer, Kurt Koffka, and Wolfgang Köhler. They aimed to move beyond behavioral atomism and understand the overall patterns of mental processes. Lewin joined the Gestalt movement and lent his own motivational slant to their program. He represented his ideas through the field concept of a "hodological space" based on the mathematics of topology. With the rise of Hitler in 1933, Lewin emigrated to the United States, holding faculty positions at such institutions as the University of Iowa and MIT. His mature works, written in America, included *Principles of Topological Psychology* and *Field Theory in Social Science*.[20]

Concepts like Lewin's can point psychology in the right direction. However, they suffer from limitations for two reasons. First, they are based entirely on numerical constructs. Second, they do not exploit all that physical field analogies might offer the mental sciences.

The structures that Einstein lauded belong to a highly flexible field subtype that deserves maximal consideration. Analogies to such special fields promise to serve the interests of psychology in a unique way by loosening the number-conserving symmetries of neutral monism during one-to-one subject–object exchanges. The properties of these fields involve invariances that are potentially more general than those on which numerical rigor is based.[21,22]

The origin of deficiencies in computer metaphors for mind lies in one-to-one restrictions on the nature of subject–object exchanges in neutral monism. One-to-one exchange explains why we know psychological facts, like the feeling of pain and its attendant bodily reactions, both subjectively and objectively. One-to-one exchange demonstrates how, in mental domains, some objective entity will correspond to every subjective concept. It thus convinces us that conscious experiences should always map into a species of matter.

However, one-to-one exchange cannot account for inverse mapping features. Donald Davidson, the Slusser Professor of Philosophy at Berkeley, has argued persuasively that while every mental and therefore intentional event is also physical, not every physical event is obviously mental.[23-25] Such reasoning must lead to doubts that any one-to-one exchange of subject and object can generate laws showing why the matter with which mind correlates always seems to be neurological.[26] That is, it cannot reveal why in nonneurological domains a subjective concept may not exist for each objective entity.

Hence, it becomes necessary to expand the one-to-one exchanges that define numbers into a more flexible maneuver, no longer rigidly bound by the one-to-one correspondence requirement of classic neutral monism. This expansion can be achieved by *restricting numerical symmetry itself* to a confined territory. Such a limit on the legitimate scope of functionalism and neutral monism will give subject–object transformations license to generate only qualified invariances, each defined independently. It will thus reduce "mind–matter" symmetries of the brain to attenuated realms. The neuropsychiatric viewpoint, in which mind and matter are treated equivalently, will thereby shrink from a "global" symmetry principle to a "local" one.

What are "global" and "local" symmetries? We may illustrate the concept of a global symmetry by returning to the simple geometric example of rotational invariance. When we turn a ball on its axis, say, 120 degrees, the ball's overall spherical shape doesn't change; it is said to exhibit symmetry during rotational transformations. Under normal circumstances, rotation of the ball entails turning each point on its surface through the same angle, 120 degrees. In such cases the symmetry is "global."[27]

However, we can modify this global rotational symmetry. If the ball is inflatable and has a skin made of pliable rubber, we might for the sake of variety try independently rotating each of several surface points a different number of degrees at the same time. To describe the resulting nonglobal invariance, structure must be added[28]; this structure is a "local" symmetry principle applied separately to each such transformation.[29] Locality represents the independence of component transformations from each other within the system.

Through locally independent rotations of different points on a ball's rubber surface, we can maintain the ball's round shape, but only at the cost of creating a web of elastic resistances. The array of such opposing forces is an example of what physicists call a gauge field. It results from global-to-local transitions in symmetry and is the special kind of field structure endorsed by Einstein. Generally, a gauge field corresponds to an abstract kind of "curvature," arising in the local divergence of any actual invariance from the ideal of some arbitrary global symmetry.[30]

Hermann Weyl (1885–1955) was the mathematician who first explicitly coined the term gauge field. He came from Hamburg, Germany, and was educated at Göttingen University, where he worked as a faculty member along with Felix Klein, David Hilbert, and others until 1913. He then moved to the Institute of Technology in Zurich, where his tenure overlapped briefly with that of Albert Einstein. Weyl finally returned to Göttingen in 1930, but left again in 1933 to protest the coming of the Third Reich. He worked at the Institute for Advanced Studies in Princeton until his retirement in 1951. Weyl's intellectual activities, while ranging over many subdisciplines within mathematics, contributed particularly to post-Newtonian physics by sharpening its concepts of fields and symmetries. The writings of Kant and other philosophers influenced his ideas.[31]

Hermann Weyl's concept of a gauge field subsumes many kinds of physical systems besides the elastic surface of a rubber ball. One such locally symmetrical structure governs electromagnetic phenomena. To understand how it works, we must first consider the global invariance of static electrical fields that have no magnetic components. Global symmetry applies to static electrical fields because their magnitudes depend only on the relative voltage difference between any two points in space and not on the absolute voltage at a single point. Hence, a static electrical field might be expected to remain invariant after transformations that raise or lower all voltages by the same amount throughout space. If the source of an electrical field moves, however, the relevant symmetry will become local; the field will not vary even if voltages at each point in space change independently by different amounts. This is because moving electrical sources generate a second force, magnetism, that balances all accounts. Magnetism and electrical forces hence add together and create a gauge field, which is the total electromagnetic interaction.[32]

An analogous gauge field governs effects that arise between interacting quantum-mechanical wavefronts. Streams of aggregated electrons can be made to undulate between positive and negative energy values at regular wave frequencies. The value at which each wave begins life at its electron emission source determines its "phase." If the source is aimed at a barrier that contains two slits, positive and negative energy values of the few waves that squeeze through either hole will add to each other at every point in space beyond the slits to produce a complex pattern. This pattern can be seen by projection onto a detector array. Changing the phase of the wavefront by the same amount at each point in space will have no effect on the additive pattern; the pattern will appear "globally symmetrical" with respect to phase shifts. If a phase-shifting device is attached to only one slit, however, the interference pattern will be altered. An identical alteration in the interference pattern will also result from placing the slits in a magnetic field; no observer could ever guess from the interference pattern change alone whether a phase-shifting device or magnet had been used. For this reason, the forces involved in both phase-shifting devices and magnets, taken together as a single entity, are said to form a gauge field lending local symmetry to the system.[33,34]

Perhaps the most famous local gauge symmetry lies in the quasi-independent physical invariances of "general" relativity theory. Relativistic global symmetries, like those causing the "twin" paradox, are restricted to small segments of time and space. These segments, like limited areas of the earth's surface viewed from our tiny human viewpoint, come close to appearing flat. The difference between what we would expect from more extensive global symmetries and what happens in the locally symmetrical world of actual space–time gives rise to gravity. It does so because relativistic space–time is "curved" by masses that attract each other.[35]

Local gauge field symmetry in its most general sense gives us a tool to surmount limits on the global invariance of one-to-one subject–object exchanges in neutral monism. It no longer matters that this kind of global symmetry cannot survive complicated relations between subjects and objects in different, independent local frames of reference. Gauge symmetry will overcome this problem by restricting the numerically self-referent invariance of neutral monism to a local domain.

Furthermore, using intentionality as a "curvature" that grounds the transition from global to local symmetry can resolve self-referent inconsistencies in numerical measurement by subordinating them to intentional concerns. This is possible because seeing intentionality as "curvature" converts semantic reference from an adjunctive property of subjective mind into its intrinsic essence.[36–40]

An analogy to ordinary geometric curvature will illustrate this last point. Curvature in geometry can be of two kinds, extrinsic and intrinsic. The extrinsic type cannot be detected by measurements obtained through means that are entirely contained within figures, like cylinders, that are affected by it. On the other hand, intrinsic curvature can be so measured.

To make the concept more concrete, we might imagine a two-dimensional surveyor doing his work in a flat, planar universe. If he picked three points, connected them with lines to form a triangle, and measured the three angles that form its vertices, he would find the sum of the angles to be 180 degrees. If his two-dimensional "universe" turned out to be the rounded lateral surface of a cylinder, the sum of angles would not change. However, if the surveyor were working within the two-dimensional outer surface of a three-dimensional sphere, the angles would add up to more than 180 degrees.

This last fact could allow the surveyor dealing with the spherical surface to conclude that his "universe" had intrinsic curvature, detectable within the confines of its own two dimensions. In contrast, the surveyor working on the cylinder would somehow have to go outside its lateral surface, into the three-dimensional space that surrounds it, in order to detect its extrinsic curvature.[41]

Gauge fields are capable of harboring intrinsic curvature. Hence, intentional gauge fields can do justice to the intrinsic, essential connection between meaning and subjective consciousness. The curvature of a gauge field will "bend" neutral monism to reflect local limits on numerical invariance and hence support an intrinsically intentional epistemology. In contrast, empirical psychologies cast meaning outside the behaving organism, attaching it to external "reinforcing" objects.[42]

The fact that subject–object relations require local symmetry and generate intentional gauge curvature is expressed in the inherent structure of the language describing them. It is easy to see that some sentences display symmetry. That is, the sense of a statement like "X is Y" may remain invariant when sentence order is reversed, exchanging the words "X" and "Y." Such sentences include "identity" assertions like "That man is John Smith."

But statements assuming the form "X is Y" can be of more than one type; they may not be assertions of identity. "Predicative" statements, for example, which make descriptive claims like "the dog is brown," also have an "X is Y" form. Symmetry does not extend to one-to-one exchanges between subject and predicate.[43] Therefore, global symmetry alone cannot subsume statements of the form "X is Y." We can handle them only by loosening global linguistic symmetry and thus turning it into a local invariance. Such generalization hinges on the verb "to be," which appears in both "identity" and "predicative" assertions.

Consider a third class of sentences in which the verb "to be" also appears: existential statements like "God is" (i.e., "God exists"). Kant pointed out that existential assertions reveal the uniquely problematic nature of "is" among linguistic constructs; existential sentences enable us to see the emptiness of "is" as an explicit, qualitatively specific predicate.[44-47] In this regard, Kant wrote that

> being is evidently not a real . . . concept . . . that can be added to the concept of a thing. . . . The small word ["is"] . . . is not an additional predicate, . . . [and does] not ascribe a new predicate to the concept.[48]

This suggests that in the framework of linguistic symmetry, we should metaphorically shrink the role of the verb "to be" down to the infinitesimal scale of "flatness" or null curvature, reducing the word "is" to negligible status. Such a readjustment requires that the relevant linguistic symmetry be local.

Kant asserted that in existential statements, the verb "to be" does have one function: It "serves to put the predicate in relation to the subject." He wrote that "if, then, I take the subject . . . and say, . . . [it] exists, . . . I only posit the subject by itself . . . as its [own] object."[49] Hence, meaningful sentences with local symmetry and significant "curvature" must substitute active verbs having *objects* in place of the verb "to be" bearing predicates. Any local symmetry generalized for a description of language, then, should link subjects not with predicates but with objects. That is to say, local linguistic symmetry will describe invariance connected with exchanges not of subjects and predicates but of subjects and objects.

꿈   꿈   꿈

Local symmetry of subject–object exchanges can help to expand our understanding of science so that it will better accommodate psychology.

Our find of scientific knowledge itself undergoes periodic growth by bursting past limits that have constrained preceding modes of thought. Philosophers of science call these limits linear ranges.[50,51] In Galileo's time, the linear range of physics included only phenomena in our everyday, earthbound environment; beyond that, to chart the paths of other planets, for example, scientists had to wait for Newton's account of changes in the force of gravity over large distances in outer space. Newton's system, in turn, had its own linear range, which limited the amount of matter that it could handle; truly massive, stellar objects required Einstein's relativity to deal with vagaries produced by strong gravitational effects.

In all these cases, creative scientists who transcended the linear limits of their own times did not regard the opening of holes in pet theories and equations as an unwelcome or paralyzing prospect. The reasoning of such scientists was productive precisely because of a weeding-out process that made room for creative improvements. "Nonlinear" science fueled intellectual progress[52] by framing its principles in ways that actually invited crises of disproof in order to advance.[53-55]

The philosopher Karl Popper (1902–   ) has given us an especially perceptive analysis of this process. Popper grew up in Vienna, where he studied physics and philosophy and heard Einstein speak in 1919. This last experience apparently influenced Popper's subsequent philosophy of science. In 1934, he published *The Logic of Scientific Discovery*, a book that turned the concept of scientific proof on its head. He subsequently settled in London, where he became a professor of logic and scientific method in 1949. In his later years, Popper extended his ideas into the domain of biology and mind through books like *Objective Knowledge* and *The Self and Its Brain* (1977). His other writings included *Conjectures and Refutations*, *The Open Society and Its Enemies*, and *The Poverty of Historicism*. He was knighted in 1965 and retired in 1969.[56-59]

Popper has shown that a good scientist will always challenge his own assumptions. His logic resembles the ancient syllogism called *modus tollens*,[60] a "taking away style" devised by the Stoic philosopher Chrysippus.[61] A Popperian scientist like Einstein keeps his antennae hungrily attuned not simply to data proving his theories, but more importantly, to potential refutation. He is eager to throw out even his favorite concepts at the moment that events show him to be wrong. A poor fit between hypothesis and experimental data, leading to the downfall of orthodox theories, will thus serve to purify his ideas and allow him to move beyond his own horizons.[62–64]

This is because, as Bronowski points out, by exploiting the intentionality of mind, the creative scientist can transcend the formalisms of numbers; he

> can go on working . . . whether the system is consistent or not. And . . . when . . . [he comes] on a profound discovery . . . which is really essentially an inconsistency in the system, then [he reorganizes] the whole thing. And that reorganization is the central act of [scientific] imagination.[65]

Scientists have this intentional capability because they are people, not mechanisms. Thus, although creative scientists always check their ideas, they do not invent their theories merely to test them mechanically. As Bronowski writes

> the test by falsification will diagnose when a theory falls sick, but it does not reflect what we ask a healthy theory to be or to do.

The reason is that

> *truth is not the only aim of science*. We want more than mere truth; what we are looking for is *interesting truth*.[66]

Any scientist who remains mired in conflicts over mere method, technique, or terminology is not serving the cause of interesting truth adequately. Syntactical form is not enough; semantic meaning is also needed. Early quantum physicists, who squabbled fruitlessly over the relative merits of two theoretical formalisms, wave and matrix mechanics, learned this very lesson in our century. Only time and attention to the similarity of their predictions revealed that the rival quantum systems housed the same semantic content in different mathematical tongues. Distinctions between matrix and wave mechanics proved to have no actual value for any scientist trying to address quantum phenomena meaningfully.

The mind of a creative scientist spawns not simple formal statements but principles with interesting meanings because intentional gauge fields weave nonlinearity into the intrinsic[67,68] structure of knowledge. An intentional gauge field hence constitutes a metastructure that is integrated with the nonlinear progression of scientific paradigms. Intentional gauge fields allow science to make adequate room for creative mental processes by subordinating numerical linearity to the intentionally nonlinear demands of conceptual progress in a natural way.[69–71] This places the numerical symmetry of neutral monism in an appropriately reduced, local perspective and frees intentionality to resonate throughout consciousness,[72,73] resolving rather than suppressing paradox.[74] Subjectively intentional windows of creativity can thereby provide routes of access to ever-increasing parts of the world outside the linear status quo of strict numerical reasoning.[75–77]

This aspect of any truly creative and humane science is crucial in psychology. It cannot be overlooked. Because gauge fields mediating the transition from global to local symmetry are nonlinear, their features cannot be mapped[78] back into an old, rigidly global reference frame without distorting their contours.

Local subject–object symmetry and its attendant intentional gauge field structure hence require the psychologist to adduce evidence not simply from numerical data but from inner subjectivity and its attendant intentional meaning as well. Only in this way can the psychologist bring his techniques into harmony with his scientific ends.[79]

9

Madness and Alienation

L ocal symmetry offers some hope for mind–body rapproche-
ment in a way that transcends the pitfalls of older philosophical models. Locally invariant principles retain the positive features
of neutral monism as a "flat" linear limit but also include nonlinear
"curvature" to make room for intrinsic intentionality. Gauge field
concepts thus get us a fair distance beyond the horizon of neuropsychiatry. However, in the form presented so far, local subject–
object symmetry still has a few inadequacies that need more
ironing out. This can be done by generalizing the concept of an
intentional gauge field yet further.

We ordinarily assume that psychological content by itself
suffices to connect mental states to the real world. As Searle points
out, we go about our everyday business quite sure that intentional
entities of the mind "are about . . . states of affairs in the world"
and that "their content directs them at these states." Moreover, we
believe that "intentional states have [real] 'conditions of satisfaction,'" and that each mental "state itself determines under what
conditions it is true . . . or . . . fulfilled." In other words, we take
it for granted that every "mental state [internally] represents its
own conditions of satisfaction."[1]

Such assumptions are not necessarily true. There is no reliable link between a subjective perception and the objective truth
of its content. We cannot discriminate illusory from real objects of

perception without engaging in flawed reasoning. Descartes himself framed the problem in clear terms when he pointed out that normal dreams can produce experiences similar to those of the "insane in their waking moments." He noted that "there are no certain indications by which we may . . . [subjectively] distinguish" dreams from reality.[2]

This dilemma relates to our epistemic gauge field model's demand that the global symmetries of neutral monism reduce simply and cleanly to a local limit. Our psychological world deviates from such neat behavior. Its complexities are harder to describe because of "singular" structures that disrupt local symmetries.

Singularities are sharp contours in fields that are otherwise smooth. Where sharp cusps exist, curvatures become infinite, the field can no longer approach the flatness of global invariance in local domains, and therefore symmetry principles no longer have any relevance.

The example of a singular cusp arising in the gravitational field theory of relativistic physics is instructive here. At the sharp apex of a physical singularity, curved space–time cannot exhibit its normal, smooth approach to the flatness of global symmetry as scales of measurement shrink. Hence, gravitational curvature increases without limit, and invariant physical laws, either global or local, cease to apply. The most notable singular entities in the physical world are the black hole and the "Big Bang."[3,4]

With intentional gauge field singularities, subject–object relations break down in similar fashion; contact between subjective mind and objective domains therefore disappears. For this reason, we can think of singularities in intentional gauge fields as representing the most severe kind of mental disturbances, psychoses.[5]

Singular psychoses arise only in the context of fields that cannot integrate "unreal" experiences with the rest of consciousness. In some instances, such harmony is not a problem. Oriental mystics have made an art out of integrating "unreal" experiences into ordinary consciousness and hence transcending the whole issue of psychosis. A few Western thinkers have attempted to move in a similar direction.[6,7] The most relentless among them was Edmund Husserl.

Husserl was born in 1859 at Prossnitz in Moravia. He learned mathematics in Berlin and Leipzig and also studied psychology under Brentano in Vienna. In 1900, Husserl became professor of philosophy at Göttingen; he moved to Freiburg in 1916 and taught there until 1929. His writings included *Logical Investigations* (1901), *Ideas for a Pure Phenomenology* (1913), *Cartesian Meditations* (1929), and *The Crisis of the European Sciences and Transcendental Phenomenology* (1935). He died in 1938 after political repression curtailed his activities.[8–11]

Husserl attempted to change Western concepts of mind by reducing the referents of intentionality to merely "immanent" objectivity. His immanent objects of consciousness included not only true but also false or even hallucinatory content.[12–16] Hannah Arendt's words expressed the idea vividly; she wrote that "though the seen tree may be an illusion, for the act of seeing it is an object nevertheless; though the dreamt-of landscape is visible only to the dreamer, it is the object of his dream."[17]

Husserl's neutral stance regarding the reality of intentional referents combined the "objective truth" of nature and the "other world" of imagination into one integrated package.[18,19] His marriage of "healthy" perception and "sick" delusion bequeathed us a natural conceptual bridge from mental health to disease.

To account for Husserl's approach in our gauge field model of mind–matter relations, we must introduce a particular structural change that integrates each psychotic singularity into its overall field environment and thus obliterates its singular status.[20] The new element that will accomplish this is called torsion.[21]

Torsion represents a kind of wobble in the integrity of a relevant local symmetry. Without torsion, we can shrink any closed path through a gauge field down to a pointlike structure. With torsion, that "point" becomes a "line" standing perpendicular to a tangent of the gauge field "surface."[22]

The difference between a torsion-free and torsional system might best be understood by way of analogy to a cork and a corkscrew. If a cork in the mouth of a wine bottle is turned without any upward or downward pressure, its depth within the neck of the bottle will not change; all point-to-point contacts between cork and glass will remain longitudinally intact. On the other hand, if the corkscrew is turned appropriately, it will withdraw the cork, smearing point-to-point contacts between cork and glass into lines. The action of turning the cork resembles a torsion-free system, while the action of the corkscrew suggests torsional effects.

Roger Penrose, the Rouse Ball Professor of Mathematics of Oxford University, has used torsion in formulating his "twistor" theory, which tries to blend the statistical uncertainties of quantum physics with the space–time structure of general relativity.[23,24] Penrose has speculated about ways in which a merger of quantum mechanics with classical relativity theory might serve to illuminate the mind–matter question.[25] His interest in the specific issues of relativistic and quantum physics is well beyond the scope of this discussion, but we might profit by appropriating his torsional perspective directly in the general service of connecting mind–matter relations to psychoses.

Twistorlike torsion conflates distinctions of size. The splaying of points into lines by torsion, like the longitudinal smearing of point-to-point contacts between cork and bottle through a corkscrew's motion, blurs boundaries between fine and coarse scale. Torsion thus maps global and local features into each other.[26] This property of torsion makes it an important adjunct to any field in which numerical magnitude has no absolute meaning. It is also this characteristic that enables torsion to integrate psychotic "singularities" into an overall field structure by obliterating the pointlike sharpness of their singular status.

             ಶ಼   ಶ಼   ಶ಼

Husserl's ontological neutrality raises questions about the existence of a "self" at the core of experience. The self's "reality" in any ontologically neutral system of thought becomes no surer than any other object's tangible existence.

Moreover, Husserl's outlook obscures the self as a consistent object in a particularly troublesome way. Husserl admits only two unwavering components to the domain of consciousness: the object of perception and its intentional meaning. The perceiver himself is relegated to an ephemeral status. The perceiving subject or "self" fades into a transitory realm that flits in and out of awareness, depending on whether consciousness at any given moment is operating unreflectively or self-reflectively.[27,28]

Husserl's thought thus underscores problems in the integrity of self-concepts. However, his ontological neutrality did not create these difficulties single-handedly. Viability of the self as a coherent idea has in fact been in trouble for over two centuries. David Hume's own ontically neutral writings started the problem by recasting reality as mere sense-data. Hume considered each of these data to be an inherently separate and distinct "atom" of perception. He deemed any causal or logical connections binding the atoms together a mere illusion. One of the traditional ways of "bundling" sense-data had been through the concept of a self as perceptual conduit. However, after Hume's atomizing of reality, selfhood along with everything else seemed to collapse into a mere "heap of perceptions." The self thus became a philosophically moribund entity.[29–31]

Kant tried to deal with this crisis by treating the self as a "transcendental" concept. That is, Kant saw the self as a thing that defies absolute logical definition but still exists in a preverbal way, providing each individual person with a continuity of thought processes over time.[32,33]

Hegel seized on the concept of time in an attempt to restore the idea of an "absolute" self. He asserted that the so-called "illogical" status of selfhood was only an artifact of Kant's limited, here-and-now perspective. Hegel tried to take in the entire span of history, which he claimed manifests the absolute self's divine evolution from internal dissonance toward total harmony. He suggested that during intermediate historical stages, the absolute, divine self will appear in partly alienated human forms.[34–36] He most likely placed Hume and Kant among these flawed forms.

Hegel's metaphysics were shaky, but they succeeded in introducing his audience to the modern concept of self-alienation. His ideas revealed that the perspective of Hume has left Western man with a blurred sense of self. Especially in our own time, when Hume's empiricism informs technical scientific practices, selfhood has been splayed over many conceptual domains and defined by none in particular. [37,38]

In psychiatry, self-alienation manifests itself most directly in the so-called "biopsychosocial model," which enjoys current popularity. This highly relativistic viewpoint claims that the self and its mind can be analyzed on many levels of scale, from molecules through organisms to whole societies. The biopsychosocial approach suggests that each level has its own legitimate properties, which augment but do not depend on those of subordinate levels. Hence, as Arthur Koestler points out in his book *The Ghost in the Machine*, human organisms become "multi-levelled hierarchies of semi-autonomous sub-wholes" as well as parts of overarching "superordinate" entities in a manner echoing Russell's theory of types. Many advocates of the biopsychosocial model use it to justify eclectic styles of psychiatric diagnosis and treatment, whose various conceptual bases nevertheless remain uncoordinated. [39,40]

Incorporating torsion within intentional gauge fields can help here. Torsional blurring merges all the different scales at which a human identifies various alienated aspects of his selfhood. In accordance with Koestler's analysis, these scales of the self include the human body's measurably physical dimensions and also two other orders of magnitude: the twin extremes of collective social phenomena and partial fragments of the self. Exclusive identification with any one or two of these three elements produces a distorted self-concept. [41] Torsion can play all three against each other, coordinate their properties of scale, and thus balance the psyche. [42]

It is important to understand exactly and concretely what somatic, collective, and fragmented identities are and how each in isolation can distort concepts of the self.

ઢ   ઢ   ઢ

Purely somatic self-identity involves obsession with one's own body. Body worship in American culture is a variant of this *idée fixe*. Neuropsychiatry in its extreme form is another example.

The warping influences of corporeal mind sets stem from humanly biased self-concepts. These are exaggerated by language, which is itself a primarily human form of mental activity.[43-46] Larger aspects of consciousness do not depend on verbal expression.[47] Only the humanly imperfect parts of our mental life find their outlets in language.[48]

A famous verbal "test" invented by Alan Turing illustrates the complementary roles of language and anthropocentrism in distorting self-identity. Turing created his "test" in an effort to decide whether computers and minds might prove equivalent. He imagined a human observer posing typewritten questions to either of two respondents hidden in separate rooms. He allowed the fictive respondents to answer only with their own typewriting. The hypothetical observer was made aware that one room contained a computer and the other a person, but did not know which room housed which respondent. Turing suggested that the crucial question was whether the human interrogator, using only his typewritten dialogues, could distinguish human from machine replies.

The Turing test seems a reasonably impersonal way to decide whether computers and minds are equivalent, until a closer look reveals that its very existence springs from the mind of a human being, Alan Turing. In this way, the circularity of human self-concepts and their verbal biases undergirds the test.

ઢ   ઢ   ઢ

Collective distortion fuses individual human self-concepts with those of some larger social entity. The wish to conform to group norms leads people to overinvest their faith in public consensus.[49-52] Language contributes to this tendency in a way that is somewhat different from its role in shaping somatic self-identity. Verbal communication by definition occurs in the public domain and thus biases its participants toward a fused mode of consciousness.[53]

George Herbert Meade (1863–1931) stands out as the thinker who most prototypically espoused the collective view of self-identity. Meade attended Oberlin College and went on for training in philosophy at Harvard and the University of Berlin. In 1891, he became a faculty member at the University of Michigan, where he fell under the influence of Charles Cooley and John Dewey. Meade moved with Dewey to the University of Chicago in 1894, eventually chairing the philosophy department there. His impact on American social psychology hence proved to be profound. Meade asserted that mental life is at bottom an adaptation to interpersonal forces, particularly communicative gestures, that shape social roles.[54,55]

Views akin to those of Meade influence modern laboratory science whose collective norms often produce a desire by researchers to seek confirmation in the work of colleagues before accepting their own experimental results as accurate. The so-called logical behaviorists have helped to codify this consensual priority. Their school of thought demands that "private" mental events of research subjects be described only in behavioral terms that are publicly verifiable.[56] Among the logical behaviorists, three prominent thinkers, Carl Hempel, Ludwig Wittgenstein, and Gilbert Ryle, merit particular comment.

The ideas of Carl Hempel grew out of logical positivism. Hempel assimilated positivistic concepts in Europe before emigrating in 1937 and then teaching at Yale and Princeton. His philosophy aimed at reducing statements about mental events to assertions about observable behavior. His efforts derived from the positivistic requirement that scientifically meaningful statements must stipulate their own "test conditions."[57–59]

Ludwig Wittgenstein's approaches are harder to pin down but no less relevant to logical behaviorism. His life and career were chaotic. He was born in Vienna in 1889 and studied engineering there. While engaged in aerodynamic research in Manchester, he met Bertrand Russell, who helped him change direction and accepted him into the philosophy department at Cambridge. Wittgenstein was plagued by depression and self-doubt, however, and left Cambridge to serve in the Austrian Army during World War I. He was captured as a prisoner of war and while interned wrote his first major philosophical treatise. After the war, he chose to work as a humble gardener, giving away a considerable estate to his sisters before returning to philosophy through a liaison with the Viennese logical positivists. He finally moved back to Cambridge in 1929 and became a professor there, albeit of an idiosyncratic kind: He never used notes for his lectures, wore no tie, took time out to live abroad in a self-constructed hut, and worked during World War II as a volunteer hospital porter. He resigned from Cambridge in 1947, traveled to Ireland and the United States, and died of cancer in 1951.

Wittgenstein's erratic philosophy changed over the years with his circumstances. Its viewpoint ranged from positivism to mysticism. However, one aspect proved highly relevant to logical behaviorism. It argued against the possibility of a "private language" originating in the nonpublic realm of mental life.[60–63] Other philosophers picked up on this concept.

The British philosopher Gilbert Ryle (1900–1976) was a colleague of Wittgenstein with allied linguistic interests. He occupied a chair as the Waynflete Professor of Metaphysical Philosophy at Oxford. Ryle claimed in his famous book of 1949, *The Concept of Mind*, that the psyche can be understood solely as publicly observable behavior if we avoid the mistake of confusing particular behavioral events with their superordinate mental categories. He attempted to "translate" subjective psychological terms into behavioral phenomena using this principle.[64–67]

Practical empirical psychologies such as J. B. Watson's behaviorism explicitly derived their rationale from the theories created by philosophers like Hempel, Wittgenstein, and Ryle. The much-vaunted "objectivity" of behaviorists really rested on collective subjectivity; for them, the final test of truth in science was agreement among scientists about empirical results.

B. F. Skinner, for example, held up "intersubjectivity" as the ultimate standard of validation for his highly mechanistic experiments. Skinner became interested in behaviorism early in life through a group of articles written by Bertrand Russell about Watson. He earned a Ph.D. in 1931 at Harvard, served on university faculties in Minnesota and Indiana, and in 1948 returned to Harvard as a professor, remaining there until 1975. He invented the Skinner Box, an apparatus that facilitated animal behavioral experiments whose results could be meticulously recorded for scientific peer review. He raised his young daughter in a criblike version of his box and set forth relevant social views in two books, *Walden Two* and *Beyond Freedom and Dignity*.[68,69] Skinner was so committed to intersubjective proof as the highest behaviorist virtue that he applied it even to learning processes in infants.[70–73]

Nationalism, class consciousness, and clique formation exemplify a side of collective thinking that is less theoretical than the ideas of Meade, Hempel, Wittgenstein, Ryle, and Skinner. Yet psychologists and psychiatrists are not immune to such social influences. Basic trends in psychiatry have been at least partly molded by social forces with origins in concrete collective domains.[74] Agendas of entire societies define much of what we call the boundaries of mental hygiene.[75–80] In our own culture, the changing situation of women has contributed to a new feminist spin on psychoanalysis. Professional athletics has created sports psychology. Ecological crises and space exploration have led to environmental psychology. Contemporary institutional demands have spawned the discipline of organizational psychology.[81]

Neuropsychiatry has followed this pattern. Neurological and numerical rigidities among today's psychologists and psychiatrists gained their first beachhead in the institutionally collective womb of modern universities. These centers of research and learning were born in nineteenth-century Germany. It was in such milieus that academic researchers like Wilhelm Wundt[82] worked to cultivate an international community of like-minded professionals.

Wundt established the first academic center for cooperative

experimental research in psychology at Leipzig in 1879. His institutionally based laboratory approach spread rapidly to other parts of Germany and to Austria, Britain, France, Holland, Belgium, Spain, and Argentina. Scholars began to interact through a multitude of new academic societies, including the *Deutsche Gesellschaft für Psychologie*, the *Société Française de Psychologie*, and the British Psychological Society. The International Congress of Psychology was inaugurated in Paris in 1889.[83,84]

Wundt's less clinically minded research students and associates,[85] who included Hall, Cattell, Scripture, Angell, Baldwin, Titchener, Witmer, Warren, Stratton, and Judd, extended his basic research methods and brought them en masse to the United States. Starting with the first American facility for experimental psychology begun by Hall in 1887 at Johns Hopkins, Wundt's approach spread across North America in less than ten years to spawn more than 20 institutionally bound psychological laboratories. In most of these new centers, empirical viewpoints, imbuing nascent researchers like Thorndike with concepts such as stimulus–response pairing, conditioning, and trial-and-error learning, pushed intersubjective bias to its limit. This process mutated Wundt's transplanted experimentalism into the pure behaviorism that came to dominate American psychology for decades.[86]

The more recent brands of computer-oriented empirical research psychology known as cognitive science have continued collective, institutional modes of operation. A symposium at MIT in 1956 formalized collective links between psychologists and information-processing theorists. By the 1980s, not only the United States but also Japan, with its Institute for New Generation Computer Technology, and Europe, with its Esprit project, were collectivizing the latest approaches of cognitive science.[87] The trend has extended into the 1990s.

In tandem with such developments, institutional interests have gained a distorting influence on the clinical practice of psychiatry. Articles in the *Psychiatric News*,[88,89] *Psychiatric Annals*,[90–92] *U.S. News and World Report*,[93] and *New York Times*[94–96] suggest that, especially in America, psychiatrists must now fight the demands of insurance companies, reviewing agencies, government departments, and a variety of private industries. As a consequence of collective institutional priorities, conformity to aggregate standards is overpowering the field of mental hygiene. The result is a "system" that values aggregate "cost-effectiveness" above all else. The quality of clinical practice is now in danger of "ratcheting down" to a level of collective mediocrity. Bureaucracies of clinical "teams," which ostensibly integrate the efforts of nurses, social workers, psychologists, and psychiatrists under "utilization managers," are paring away autonomous professionals and investing the herd with increasing clinical authority.

Patients suffer as a consequence of these facts. Already, alienating institutional imperatives have led to the collective treatment of patients as mere categories, while individual interests get short shrift. Institutional entities block private utilization of many resources; more and more, regulatory obstacles deny patients prolonged hospitalization, personalized custodial care, long-term psychotherapy, and experimental drugs.[97–102] Institutional policies also increasingly subvert the personal intimacy of the doctor–patient relationship, choking and degrading one-on-one psychotherapeutic efforts.

❧   ❧   ❧

The third variety of self-distortion, fragmentation, splinters the total human individual into separate pieces and hence artificially isolates selected faculties of each potentially whole mind. Cognitive neuroscience provides an example through its concept of specialized mental "modules," each with a different function dedicated, for instance, to memory or spatial perception.[103–106]

Here, too, language plays a role. In the modern technical world, esoteric jargon intelligible only to specialists[107] dominates our verbal life. Jargon warps words to serve only limited practical goals, not general exploratory imperatives. Each isolated component of the resulting splintered lexicon takes as its intentional content just those concrete objects useful in satisfying fixed desires and appetites.[108–118]

Technical language thus splits the free curiosity of whole selves into linguistically compartmentalized functions with different, limited vocabularies in different areas of discourse.[119–121] An exclusion principle segregates the self's parts, verbally atomizing their mutual coherence into discrete subcomponents.[122] The specialized and distorted contents of each component are then each reified in isolation.[123] Mental life hence disintegrates into a tower of Babel dividing and degrading inquisitive personalities into specialized self-caricatures.

Modern technical "science" carries these trends into the laboratory. There, it trades open exploration for the chance merely to manipulate nature.[124] Marcuse outlined in detail how technical perspectives "*a priori*" reduce the natural world to mere objects of control by fragmented practical imperatives. He attributed this property of technological pseudoscience to its fetishistic exactness.[125] Limits imposed by control parameters "operationalize" technical experiments into inflexibly tight designs that serve the needs and intent of an investigator's pragmatically[126] oriented aims. Thus technical science by its very nature becomes "systematic anticipation and projection . . . in accordance with the measurable power to be extracted" from its objects of study.[127]

Since World War II, professorial slots throughout American universities have accommodated more and more academicians who fit the technical mold. Such scholastic technicians can turn into myopic pedants, each under pressure to pursue his own parochial field of expertise. Consequently, without real dialogue, the broader currents of free inquiry in the academic world may narrow into piecework-style laboratory research.[128–133]

Psychiatry's own technology, jargon, and training methods have come to foster overspecialization, fracturing the psychiatric personality into a species of the modern academic pseudoself. By the time many candidates in psychiatry enter their residency, the range of theoretical perspectives available to them has already dwindled to a single technical approach; fatal defects in medical education ensure bias against less "rigorous" viewpoints.[134] For premedical college students, some of whom are destined for psychiatric careers, required courses largely exclude the humanities. In medical schools themselves, basic science curricula are almost entirely compiled by biologists, whose teaching neglects perspectives less precise than their own.[135]

The shrinkage of conceptual choices in psychiatric training is now worsening as some academics advocate formal abandonment of all nontechnical outlooks in psychiatric residency programs. There is a strong recent push to codify this parochialism.[136] Such a change would leave little room to nurture young clinicians in the broader aspects of their chosen field.

Even seasoned psychiatrists, schooled in more old-fashioned and less technically restrictive styles, feel the pressure of professional self-fragmentation. "Utilization management," a recent mandate for bureaucratic overseers to review decisions made by clinicians, unloads a deluge of pragmatically reified demands on modern psychiatry. It formulates criteria for the desirability of various clinical practices according to their perceived effectiveness in satisfying specific aims. First among these aims is the elimination of a patient's "danger to himself or to others."[137] Toward the end of keeping mental health care within the functional bounds of "medical necessity," the mind set of utilization management thus creates highly concrete standards for weighing pragmatic psychiatric choices.[138–141]

The result is a linearly algorithmic approach to diagnostic workups, psychotherapeutic interventions,[142–144] hospital admissions, and even the clinical applicability of different theoretical models. Officially proposed guidelines aim to spell out specific dicta regarding treatment of eating disorders, schizophrenia, bipolar illnesses, geriatric diseases, outpatient evaluations, and inpatient treatments. Meanwhile, the bureaucratic efforts of utilization management's monitoring agents enforce conformity of psychiatric practice to preferred "profiles" and curtail deviations from officially sanctioned outcomes. Imposed, pragmatically delimited imperatives thus drive psychiatrists to focus on quick fixes in the name of measurable efficacy.[145–151]

If all such trends come to fruition, the wholeness of the psychiatrist's creative self will be smothered instead of nourished by his work. Clinical efforts, once sources of creativity, will shrivel completely into the meaningless, piecemeal drudgery of protocols and prescriptions.

Moreover, everyone will suffer for it. The consequences will rebound especially into the lives of patients. Self-fragmentation implicit in technical models of the psyche will provide excuses for psychiatrists to cut away many therapeutic avenues that would otherwise be available. Reified concepts, having already split the self into mental modules,[152–154] developmental "stages," and "atomic" behaviors,[155,156] will reduce all patients to objects of controlled, experimental behavioral scrutiny.[157] Patient populations will completely degenerate into groups of guinea pigs that are either "relevant" or "unentitled" to particular specialized clinical procedures.[158]

ᴈ☙   ᴈ☙   ᴈ☙

We do not necessarily have to perceive ourselves as slaves of the somatic, collective, or fragmenting self-distortions elaborated above. As the philosopher Donald Palmer points out, our self-concepts depend only on our chosen "picture of the self," and "no believable account corresponds to one or another of these pictures" exclusively.[159]

Torsion, applied to intentional gauge field theory, may offer the possibility of correcting warped restrictions in our thinking. A novel, balanced, liberating perspective,[160] stemming from a three-fold symmetry of self-scales compatible with torsion, might thereby transcend any single view of the self. In this respect, torsional approaches jibe with self-exploratory schools of psychotherapy that try to integrate the various modes of self-alienation. Ego therapies attempt to heal the fragmenting split between mind and body and between different compartmentalizations of unconscious mental life. Existential therapies, like those of Reich, Gestaltists, and "body-work" advocates, try to integrate the total human being, including his mind and body. "Transpersonal" therapies address the collective level of self-identity.[161]

Some existing models might even be said to anticipate the need for meshing all three scales.[162] An expanded, three-dimensionally balanced, intentional gauge field with torsional features could focus these nascent models into a new understanding of mind. The concept of the self might be integrated by this way of connecting and balancing all the different alienated levels of scale in a single symmetry principle. Numerical aspects of the symmetry could be handled legitimately as long as all relevant component transformations remained independent.

Modern physicists have already developed methods of dealing with phenomena that fluctuate among different orders of magnitude. One mode of attack is the so-called "renormalization block-spin lattice" approach, which allows analysis of magnetic changes in matter undergoing temperature variations near a critical value.[163,164]

A more relevant method involves concepts of supersymmetry. This approach tries to unify the forces of nature by recasting the two overall categories of known subatomic particles, bosons and fermions, as different, superficial aspects of an underlying superparticle. The superparticle is specified in a way that leaves its basic operating principles invariant whether it appears as a boson or a fermion.

Bosons are governed by Bose–Einstein statistics, which make the particles aggregate in coherent collective states. This renders their properties somewhat similar to the behavior of collectively alienated selves. Fermions, on the other hand, are governed by Fermi–Dirac statistics. Their behavior tends toward mutual exclusion of the sort exhibited by components of fragmenting self-alienation.

We might consider adapting the idea of supersymmetry to psychology by setting up a gauge invariance involving the collective and fragmented scales of self-alienation on the basis of exchanges between Bose–Einstein and Fermi–Dirac statistics. This strategy would address the fungibly "extensive" and frangibly "intensive" aspects of self-scale. Completing the symmetry in a psychological domain would also require a third element that accounts for somatic self-alienation. We might well assign to that scale an everyday, commonsense mode of statistics named after the nineteenth-century scientists James Clerk Maxwell, Josiah Willard Gibbs, and Ludwig Boltzmann.

Traditional concepts of number, even if reduced from a global to a local invariant, may not fit into this enhanced scheme. We must be open to alternative invariants that demand changes in our definition of numbers themselves. For example, quaternions might prove appropriate.

The great Irish mathematician William Rowan Hamilton (1805–1866) discovered quaternions. He was a genius who had shown evidence of intellectual precocity at the age of three and mastered several foreign languages by his tenth year. At 12, Hamilton met a famed prodigy in arithmetical calculation, Zerah Colburn, who introduced him to mathematics. By the age of 17, Hamilton had made several new mathematical discoveries, and as a student at Trinity College his worth became recognized. At the age of 22, he was appointed professor of astronomy at his alma mater. Hamilton then proceeded to revolutionize the quantitative study of light and to create a new mathematical language for Newton's physics that paved the way for quantum mechanics in the next century. Yet with all these accomplishments, Hamilton considered his discovery of quanternions the peak of his career.[165]

To understand the nature and possible psychological relevance of quaternions, it is instructive first to consider the idea of a "vector." Quantum physicists depend on two-dimensional vectors whose dual components behave like mutually perpendicular arrows. Scientists assign these arrows probability "amplitudes" whose individual lengths they cannot directly measure. This inaccessability of raw vector data to direct measurement creates a degree of symmetry absent from everyday space: Only the summed "squares" of paired vector amplitudes furnish real, measurable probability values.

If we expand this construct into a cubic version, the resulting three-pronged vectors and their rotational properties can be described by the entities called quaternions. These are not numbers in the usual sense, though they often contain "impure" elements that behave like standard numbers.

Gauge invariance of a quaternionic self-representation might allow torsion to distribute symmetry among the three scales of alienated identity, recast as analogues of Bose–Einstein, Fermi–Dirac, and Maxwell–Gibbs–Boltzmann statistics. A fully symmetrical, three-dimensionally vectored approach could then purge any asymmetries involving traditional numerical concepts.

Quaternions might therefore also provide a rigorous yet intentionally potent way of understanding psychotic phenomena. They could accomplish this by integrating the singular properties of psychoses into torsional structures more comprehensive than a gauge field with simple numbers as local invariants.[166–175]

10

Broken Symmetries of the Neuropsychiatric Marketplace

The desire to find a physical basis for mental illness has been around since ancient times. However, it has grown into an obsession only over the last 150 years. This timing coincides with the development of modern capitalist economies.[1–3]

We therefore should not be surprised to find a hidden link joining the theoretical bases of biological psychiatry and economic thought. Neither should it shock us to learn that the profit motive and its compulsive attachment to "cost-effectiveness" are increasingly skewing the mental health profession toward biotechnology and neuroscience. CAT scans and medication regimens appear to consume less time and labor than empathy and psychotherapeutic dialogue; hence, we can expect trends toward neurotechnology in psychiatric care to continue.[4,5]

It makes sense to seek the nature of the fundamental link between neuropsychiatry and economics in order to address its attendant problems. This line of inquiry, as we will see, ultimately points back to the issue of torsion in intentional gauge fields. However, full understanding also requires us first to become at least somewhat familiar with the history of economic thought.

In the Middle Ages, most people lived in a feudal system based on religious tradition and stable social relationships. Worldly wealth had less value than heavenly salvation.[6] Hence, feudal societies bogged down in the hardest and most drawn-out productive methods. Trade was limited to local markets, advertising was banned, and the abstract concepts of modern economics (land, labor, and capital) remained irrelevant.[7,8]

The first national market system was born in seventeenth-century Britain.[9] It appeared because of nascent secularism, a burgeoning drive for scientific innovation,[10] and new means of transport that facilitated long-distance commercial transactions.[11]

Economics as a modern, quantitative discipline arose at about this time. Its author was William Petty (1623–1687), an Oxford University physician and anatomist. Petty's book, *Political Arithmetick*, introduced ideas like the division of labor, monopolies, and price–value distinctions.[12]

Adam Smith (1723–1790) refined Petty's concepts. He also introduced his own new theories and earned a reputation as the first great economist.

Smith was Scottish and attended Glasgow University, where he became professor of logic and moral philosophy. He went on to tutor royalty and live in Paris, which afforded him the chance to meet Voltaire, a social thinker of great renown. In 1767, Smith returned to Britain and published his famous economic work, *An Inquiry into the Nature and Causes of the Wealth of Nations*. He moved to Edinburgh in 1778 to take up duties as Commissioner of Customs.[13,14]

The market as conceived by Smith existed to serve consumers, whose appetites determined avenues of production.[15] Smith felt that consumer priority was essential in providing a moral basis for market economies.[16]

Smith also asserted that it is "human nature to barter and exchange."[17] He believed that consumer priority and the human propensity to trade combined to create predictable economic laws. These "laws" were analogies to the Newtonian paradigm, which had recently scored impressive successes in the field of physics.

Smith's economic version of Newton's laws predicted that freedom of individuals to act in the interests of their own greed, like selfish atoms in a market-oriented universe, would beget overall collective prosperity.[18,19]

Smith's understanding, however, was static; the intrusion of novel economic factors immanent in the coming Industrial Revolution did not play a role in his thinking.[20] He was able to foresee mechanization of labor,[21] but he could not predict the misery that factory life would inflict on workers.

Thomas Malthus (1766–1834) and David Ricardo (1772–1823) possessed a later vantage point that gave them a much more pessimistic outlook than Smith. Both made dire prophesies based on the poverty rife in the England of their day. Malthus predicted that since human populations always increase more rapidly than their food supply, Smith's model of prosperous social equilibrium was doomed to failure. Ricardo made analogous statements derived from a consideration of farm rents.

In the long run, the forecasts of neither Malthus nor Ricardo panned out. They failed to anticipate that with industrial advances, families would come to desire fewer offspring and technology would increase the food yield from each unit of land.[22,23]

By the nineteenth century, economic distribution in industrialized countries like England had become more equitable. Saving money therefore became possible for more people,[24] and Smith's idea of consumer priority gained ever wider currency through cooperative movements connected to Britain's Labour Party.[25] Distribution rather than production of goods became the most contentious economic issue. John Stuart Mill (1806–1873) articulated this trend. He drew a sharp distinction between production, whose technical limits defined his view of economics, and distribution, which he felt was merely an issue for political debate. His economic dualism led to a split between quantitative, "neoclassical" economics and "metaeconomics." That schism has not healed to this day.[26,27]

The neoclassical camp came to dominate Western economic thinking. Its members spread the quantitative method of analyzing supply and demand throughout Europe and North America. Yet, as they worked, unexpected anomalies that confounded their predictive calculations kept cropping up. Unemployment, colonial exploitation, short-term depressions, and long-term growth slowdowns appeared in contexts that demanded new thinking. Some economists coped by tacking addenda on to existing models. Others looked for completely novel approaches.

Alfred Marshall (1842–1924) addressed the question of extended economic trends by distinguishing the short-term value of a commodity from the long-term cost of producing it. In his thinking, Marshall used a concept of evolution toward equilibrium[28] that was connected to old quasi-Newtonian assumptions about supply and demand.[29] Dissenters were quick to point out the inconvenient monkey wrench of disequilibrium-producing upheavals like war and revolution.[30]

John A. Hobson (1858–1940) tried to analyze the issues of both unemployment and colonialism. He argued that piled-up savings by the rich had bled the poor of England and drained away consumer demand. The wealthy were thus driven to acquire and invest in overseas colonies, where fresh demand existed.[31]

John Maynard Keynes (1883–1946) attacked the problem of economic depression. He saw it as a result of divided labor, with financial specialists handling savings apart from investment.[32] Keynes asserted that this segregation led to mismatches, producing cyclical economic disasters.[33] He saw a role for government in taking up periodic slack to "prime the pump" of effective investment.[34]

None of these thinkers came up with a durable solution to economic crises, which have recurred even in our own time. Moreover, each crisis seems to have grown out of situations not foreseen by prior theories. Financial disasters and economic theories have leapfrogged over each other, with innovations in theory never quite catching up to phenomena in the marketplace.

The metaeconomic camp, whose name was coined by E. F. Schumacher,[35] responded to this situation by trying to explain financial debacles in radical terms. Many of its members adopted

approaches that questioned the very soundness of economics itself as a discipline. Metaeconomic critics included Max Weber,
Karl Marx, Thorstein Veblen, Joseph Schumpeter, Herbert Marcuse, and Erich Fromm.[36] The views of several are especially
relevant to this discussion.

Max Weber was born in 1864 into the family of a Reichstag
member in Germany. He grew up in Berlin in a home where
prominent political figures of Bismarck's capital were frequent
guests. Weber attended the Universities of Berlin, Göttingen,
Strasbourg, and Heidelberg, studying economics, history, law,
and philosophy. He joined the university faculties in Heidelberg
and Freiburg as an economist, but his work became more famous
among sociologists. He died in 1920.

Weber's most important book was *The Protestant Ethic and the
Spirit of Capitalism*. In it he set forth the idea that today's economic
market practices derive not only from modern techniques of
production. Weber claimed that above and beyond any material
factors promoting capitalist development, the sense of a religious
"calling" to entrepreneurial activity has helped spawn the modern
businessman. Historical sources for this concept are rooted in the
belief systems of seventeenth-century Protestant sects like Calvin-
ism, with its emphasis on the value of self-denying work, thrift,
and their fruits as signs of Divine grace.[37–39]

Weber also suggested that the modern cultural perspective
nurtured by capitalism involves a distorting "rationalization" and
"mathematization" of the world that is reflected in division of labor
and bureaucracy. This insight was picked up by later theorists.[40]

Thorstein Veblen, another important metaeconomist, was
born in 1857 and grew up in rural Wisconsin and Minnesota.
Veblen earned a doctorate in philosophy in 1884 at Yale and then
served as a professor in the Midwest, at Stanford University, and at
the New School for Social Research. His unorthodox anthropological approach to economics, personal nonconformity, sexual
adventures, and agnosticism prevented him from enjoying un-
qualified academic acceptance. However, he published such important books as the *Theory of the Leisure Class* and the *Theory of*

Business Enterprise. He died in 1929, having accurately predicted the coming of a second world war.[41]

Veblen identified the activities of the upper or "leisure" classes in our society as nonproductive and parasitic on the manual labor of less advantaged groups. He based this concept on comparisons to behaviors in primitive tribal cultures. He showed that upper-class status is always displayed by conspicuously wasteful consumption and that striving among lower classes for the ability to live and consume like the upper class lends stability to social norms.[42] For Veblen, the disutility of this wasteful consumption and its ineluctable growth[43] betrayed a subterranean irrationality in economic life.[44]

Joseph Schumpeter (1883–1950) was another incisive metaeconomic thinker. His career encompassed professorships in Europe and at Harvard, a stint as Minister of Finance in post–World War I Austria, and the authorship of several books, including *Capitalism, Socialism, and Democracy*.

Schumpeter focused on the diminishing role of risk and adventure in the entrepreneurial spirit.[45] He showed that modern technological innovation has changed capitalists from entrepreneurs into managers. Employers have moved in this bureaucratic direction in order to retain power that would otherwise flow toward the engineers who run their increasingly automated plants.[46] The process has elevated caution above risk in capitalist enterprise and suppressed the aggressively innovative character seen in earlier businessmen.[47] It has also created giant corporate and government entities whose size allows them to manipulate demand through advertising.[48]

Karl Marx (1818–1883) was by far the most important and provocative metaeconomist. Marx was born into a comfortable bourgeois German Jewish family that converted to Protestantism. He began legal studies at the University of Bonn at the age of 17, but ran into trouble because of rowdy conduct and drunkenness; his father forced his transfer to the University of Berlin. There, against paternal wishes, Marx became a student not of law but of philosophy. He joined the Young Hegelian movement and earned his doctorate in 1841. His political radicalism sabotaged ambitions for a university appointment and pushed him into journalism. His criticism of government policy and party affiliations in Cologne and Paris led to expulsion from those cities. However, during these travails, in 1844 Marx managed to produce his first substantial political tract, the *Economic and Philosophic Manuscripts*, and in 1845 he wrote another book, *The Holy Family*. Marx then moved to Brussels with his wife, child, and new associate, Friedrich Engels. There he wrote works including *The German Ideology* and *The Poverty of Philosophy*. He also visited England and joined the London-based Communist League, for whom he and Engels composed *The Communist Manifesto* in 1848. In the same year, the Belgian government forced Marx and his family out of Brussels. Political changes elsewhere forced him to wander until 1849, when he settled in London. He then renewed ties with the Communist League, produced several lesser monographs, and began a life-long project, the writing of his three-volume masterwork, *Das Kapital*. He obtained tenuous financial support for himself, his wife, and their six children through Engels's family business connections in Manchester. He endured ongoing poverty and the death of several children before finding work writing for a foreign newspaper. He finally earned recognition from other, like-minded revolutionaries and lived to see the published part of *Das Kapital* translated into Russian.[49–51]

Marx is best known for creating revolutionary doctrines that led to the horrors of Soviet Communism.[52] It is true that his flawed prescriptions for curing the ills of capitalism failed miserably. However, his diagnoses were another matter. They showed him to be a psychologically astute analyst of life in market economies. He practiced metaeconomics in the same way that Freud created meta-psychology: He looked behind the facade of standard paradigms to plumb the unconscious motives that lead us to think paradigmatically in the first place.[53] Marx probed beneath the surface elements of economic theory and investigated hidden ideological sources buried deep in the history of capitalism.[54]

Despite the profundity of his analyses, Marx was not recognized as a psychological thinker. Most likely, this paucity of recognition stemmed from his lack of formal training in psychology, his enthusiasm for violent political methods, and the fact that many of his psychologically relevant works were not published until well after he died.[55]

Marx produced his metaeconomic insights by borrowing Hegel's rarified, crypto-theological concept of psychological self-alienation and adapting it to the workaday realm of economic discourse.[56,57] Marx claimed that ideas arise not from some absolute, divine spirit but from the context of their worldly environment.[58] He therefore asserted that human alienation has evolved over the course of history because of changes in modes of mundane economic production. He saw the social "dialectic" of class antagonisms as the driving engine of such change.[59]

Marx understood the flow of historical time in terms of economic stages. In his view the latest stage was capitalism, through which human labor, both physical and mental, had become maximally "alienated" into an exploited commodity.[60,61]

He singled out labor as a special kind of commodity. Marx considered all commodities to be "social heiroglyphics," encoding in fluctuations of their economic value the prior history of capitalist society.[62] He agreed with economists since Aristotle that the value of any commodity has two determinants: its intrinsic material utility and its value as an item to be exchanged.[63] However, Marx alone saw labor as a peculiar commodity with a value that generates a surplus when "consumed" by an employer.[64]

Marx interpreted the introduction of industrial machinery as a way for employers competing with other capitalists to cut their labor costs. Yet he also recognized that over the long haul, automation would work against business owners by reducing the "surplus" value of labor in their employ.[65] Moreover, machinery would bring with it a harmful assembly-line mentality that could estrange workers from the products of their own creative efforts.[66]

This "alienation" of labor is a reality. It drains the creative energy of the worker into compulsive drudgery for the benefit of another person, his employer, who becomes the social embodiment of the worker's own self-estrangement.[67] It also isolates the employer from his own humanity by externalizing his notion of self into money and acquisitive greed.[68] Alienation of both worker and employer creates waste[69] and worsens as competition among businesses drives them to saturate more and more of their operations with the latest technology.[70,71] It leads to a "false consciousness" in which commercially oriented prejudices determine all thought, reducing even intellectual life to a mere marketplace of technical ideas.[72]

Orthodox Marxists have perverted or buried many of these concepts. The practices of Communist regimes have mocked the idea of alienation with particular irony. However, a group of Western metaeconomists called the Frankfurt School has pushed some of Marx's best work forward and used it to develop new insights.

The Frankfurt School began in connection with the Institute for Social Research. The institute was founded in 1923, through private funding by a grain merchant, Felix Weil, as the first university-affiliated Marxist research center in Germany.

During the tenure of the first director, Carl Grunberg, the institute's journal published work of both an empirical and a theoretical nature. Although its members included German Communist Party members from that era, others also worked there, and an eclecticism missing in most Marxist organizations prevailed.

When Max Horkheimer replaced Grunberg in 1930, metaeconomic thinkers like Herbert Marcuse, Erich Fromm, Theodor Adorno, and Horkheimer himself began publishing works in a new periodical, the *Journal of Social Research*. Their writings attempted to revise and update Marxist critiques of capitalism. The goal was to incorporate ideas outside orthodox Marxism, such as Hegelian idealism, psychoanalysis, existentialism, phenomenology, and the concepts of Max Weber, in order to account for new developments in the West and the malignant turn taken by Soviet Communism in Russia. The result was a range of related viewpoints subsumed under the general category of "critical theory."

Since most members of the Frankfurt School were political radicals, Hitler's rise to power in 1933 forced them to flee Germany. Horkheimer and Adorno settled in California, jointly wrote a book portraying empirical science as a repressive ideology, and finally moved back to Frankfurt after World War II in order to restart their institute. German successors like Jurgen Habermas, Oskar Negt, and Alfred Schmidt carried on the work of Horkheimer and Adorno and added their own unique contributions to the movement.

Some emigré members of the Frankfurt School, like Herbert Marcuse and Erich Fromm, never returned to Germany. Marcuse in particular remained in New York and became famous as the "father" of the New Left in the 1960s and 1970s. He was also awarded university chairs at Brandeis and in San Diego. His critiques exposed the power of modern capitalism in a "totally administered society" to invade and control even noneconomic aspects of life, thwarting any chance for internal reform. His analyses also incorporated Freud's concept of a "death instinct" into critical social theory, putting a distinctly Marcusian spin on neo-Marxist thought. Marcuse's works included *Hegel's Ontology and the Theory of Historicity* (1932), *Reason and Revolution* (1941), *Eros and Civilization* (1955), *Soviet Marxism* (1958), *One-Dimensional Man* (1964), *An Essay on Liberation* (1969), *Counterrevolution and Revolt* (1972), and *The Aesthetic Dimension* (1979).[73-77]

❧   ❧   ❧

Metaeconomics in all the forms outlined above can serve as background to help us understand the connection between money, neurotechnology, and the current state of psychiatry. That tie-in is related to the local threefold symmetry among somatic, collective, and fragmented scales of alienated self-identity discussed in Chapter 9.

The symmetry of self-scales as we have formulated it is helpful but if wrongly expressed in standard numerical terms can produce flaws. The pertinent defects may be visualized as a series of crimps that limit torsion within intentional gauge fields. Each "crimp" has the effect of ensuring that a torsional state will fail to reflect the full threefold symmetry of its underlying field. Components of the symmetry will still be present, but torsional skewing of the system will hide their full expression.[78,79]

Analogy to a Ping-Pong ball under stress illustrates this principle in a different setting. The ball, if compressed by a uniform force distributed over its entire surface, will dimple at one point. Some spherical symmetry thus will be lost. However, rotations around the axis passing through the dimple will remain symmetrical. The full invariance will be "broken," though some element of symmetry will persist.[80]

Because the whole three-dimensionally invariant web of self-identity tends to "break" apart when suffused by defective torsion, symmetry relations between different scales of alienation unravel. In particular, the soma splits off from collective and fragmented self-distortions. However, the process of symmetry-breaking spares and preserves invariances involving only the twofold subgroup of collective and fragmented self-identity scales.[81,82] These two modes of alienation thus come to complement each other as interchangeable elements of a nonorientable, compound pseudoselfhood.

Let us call this compound pseudoselfhood "normative" identity. It creates a delusory equivalence between the private and public worlds, making all the fragmented motives and desires of the self seem, in Marcuse's words, to "issue from and re-enter a societal ensemble."[83]

Such normative distortion turns technique into an alienating instrument of conformity.[84,85] Normative motives root themselves in remote, intersecting fragments permuted by social conditions.[86–92] The personal standards of the self cease to flow from private sensibilities, goals become communal, and all agendas subordinate themselves to the technical demands of the social status quo.[93]

Normed selves thereby mutate into interchangeable instruments[94] of each other's appetites. They hence support our market-oriented world view, bequeathed by Adam Smith, according to whom it is "human nature to barter and exchange."[95] This outlook leads naturally to the related technical notion that measurable "use values," stemming from fragmented private motives, and "exchange values," deriving from interpersonal commerce,[96–101] are linked through economic commodities. The concept is a quantitative one consistent with our exaggerated contemporary fetish for numbers.[102]

Quantitative economics provides a vehicle by which the normative social science of Adam Smith can appropriate the modern prestige of mathematical logic. Marcuse notes that our enthusiasm for numbers thus makes the fungible "social position of the individual in his relations to others appear . . . determined by objective qualities and laws, . . . calculable manifestations of (scientific) rationality."[103] This leads in normative social theories to a modern replacement of the older "personal dependence (of the slave on the master, the serf on the lord of the manor, the lord on the donor of the fief, etc.) with dependence on the 'objective order of things' (on economic laws, the market, etc.)."[104] Such economic "laws" include supposedly "quantifiable qualities" of human economic interaction such "as units of abstract labor power, calculable in units of time."[105] They also include money, its exchange, and the interest it spawns.[106]

Economic concepts like these are built into our culture. Market-oriented ideas including the labor theory of value, price–value distinctions, division of labor, and mechanized production have seeped from the minds of seminal economists like Petty and Smith into the mass prejudices of our society as a whole.[107] Market-oriented norms of self-identity, whether shaped by advertising, heroic myths of the entrepreneur, or the seductive inducements of material prosperity, promote uncompromising pecuniary priorities. The resulting biases cast all people as equally self-seeking market components that together fuel aggregate economic growth.

This ideologically driven view of all people as mere economic vendors and consumers has wormed its way into modern American medical practice through incursions of third-party insurers with their cost-conscious agendas. It has allowed the bottom line of a ledger sheet to replace patient welfare as an "ethical" end. Medical free-marketeers, including purveyors of mental health care for pure profit, are thus committed to understand health delivery only from the perspective of soulless competition. They have directed doctor–patient interfaces toward an arena of ubiquitous greed that some economists suppose begets overall economic productivity. Hence, medical care, including biologically oriented psychiatric services, has come to be regarded as a concrete material commodity through which, according to the shopworn dogma of Adam Smith, both seller and buyer support the general market by pursuing their own private interests.[108]

Federal action, including a combination of decisions by the Federal Trade Commission and the Supreme Court, has encouraged this kind of inappropriately competitive approach in a traditionally noncommercial profession. In addition, a dramatic rise in the number of medical practitioners has helped to make market-oriented competition the prevailing mode by which physicians provide care to patients. As a result, "for-profit" hospitals and clinics have proliferated, and these facilities calculate the aliquots of care that they dole out to patients according to financial formulae.[109] Impending health care "reforms" guided by principles of "managed competition" promise to pay no less homage than the present system to such priorities.

Areas of medicine affected by market-oriented ideologies include psychiatry. Most private psychiatric hospitals are now investor-owned.[110] Moreover, today's proponents of public funding in psychiatry often rely on financial arguments, measuring the social costs of mental illness in dollars, to justify allocating money for research.[111]

Nevertheless, we must bear in mind that the idea of an abstract economic "mechanism" governing any "market," including psychiatry, is just a normative delusion. As Schumpeter understood, manipulation of consumer demand by advertisers and not the "invisible hand" of impersonal market forces runs much of the commerce in today's society.[112]

Advertising promotes consumption, which many of today's leading economists regard as the optimal basis for measuring our "standard of living." Such a slant discourages us from seeing any difference between worthwhile and worthless consumption. Propaganda derived from norms based on economically fungible selves extolls the conspicuously wasteful consumption noted by Veblen. Advertising pushes even destructive consumption, including practices that degrade the environment. Our culture convinces us that we must "live and die . . . productively" with waste as the "price of progress" in the conduct of all our business.[113–117]

Many mental health professionals today unwittingly embrace this view and invest themselves in cheerless compulsive work,[118] driven less by creative joy than by remuneration or hierarchical advancement. This approach inevitably produces more wheel-spinning than progress. One result is a deluge of insignificant research papers and a distressing "tendency for the subject to sprawl and to pile up accumulations of not very significant detail."[119]

If mounting irrelevancies distract the attention of academic researchers, they also divert clinical psychiatric resources away from authentically self-exploratory enterprises. Instead, priority is often given to therapeutic techniques that are "cost-effective" in the short term but may have no lasting significance.

Such diversions, along with other medical market excesses that include psychiatric activities, palpably damage American health care delivery in general and mental health in particular. According to Arnold Relman, former editor of the *New England Journal of Medicine*, a number of hospitals and clinics throughout the country wastefully serve their own bottom line rather than needy segments of their home communities. Some ostensibly provide unnecessary services to wealthy patients for inflated returns, while obstacles deny "utilization" of resources for poor people. Certain physicians reportedly invest in facilities to which they refer their own patients. Others apparently arrange with drug wholesalers to sell discounted products to patients for profit. A few medical researchers allegedly receive inducements to test and tout particular products, often produced by corporations in which the scientists themselves own stock. All in all, a Congresswoman investigating the situation has estimated that 160 billion dollars, or 20 percent of all health care expenditures in 1991, derived from fraud or other questionable practices.[120–122]

Psychiatric segments of the medical market seem to have participated in such waste. The *Psychiatric News*[123] relates that some investor-owned hospital chains specializing in mental health care have actively pursued policies of high-pressure marketing and employee incentive structures in order to fill all their beds with paying patients regardless of medical need.

Meanwhile, the growth of compulsive work habits among psychiatrists helps shape official definitions of mental "illness" to include the inability to sustain disciplined labor.[124] One might worry that eventually even those merely questioning the value of compulsive work will be labeled as disturbed. In that case critics in the tradition of Weber, Veblen, and Marx, who have gone beyond economics in their meta-analyses of alienated drudgery,[125] could soon find themselves with psychiatric diagnoses.

Purveyors of the modern economic bias toward mindless work and consumption do not take kindly to exposure of its destructive side, which they hide under the "value-free" lexicon of cost–benefit analysis.[126] This sort of language, according to Marcuse, converts the consumer-oriented norms of our whole culture into "a veil of symbols which [both] represents and at the same time masks . . . the world of [perverse economic] practice."[127] Our society with its economic apologists is therefore able to suppress opposition to its market ideology by invoking cost–benefit arguments that seemingly reduce critiques of the market to wild-eyed, "utopian" speculation.[128]

Economically driven behavior hence "tends to become the stuff of . . . [self-justifying] administration."[129] In the psychiatric world of which American medicine is a part, administrative absorption of professional autonomy through financial leverage plays itself out with a special vengeance. A number of authors[130–142] have described the resulting sorry situation. According to them, 24 investor-owned companies controlled 80 percent of all clinical psychiatric hospital beds as of June 1992. In addition, a giant, interlocking national grid of shared risk now backs up third-party payment programs throughout the United States. Bureaucratic tentacles of utilization management by insurers are invading progressively larger segments of clinical psychiatric practice. It has been estimated that by 1995, more than four fifths of all private mental patients will fall under the purview of managed care. In this way, such controls as practice guidelines will come to dominate psychiatry completely. "Gatekeepers" operating from a standardized cookbook will assume all triage powers. Utilization management will then expand from inpatient into other sectors of psychiatric practice. Managed competition reforms may actually accelerate these trends.

Stifling administrative interests are controlling not only clinical psychiatry. They also direct both public and private institutional subsidies of medical research. Research bureaucracies draw their strength from the marketplace of ideas through which their technical goals attract the collectively empowered financial support of uncultivated mass constituencies. This gives the popular will a grim but real advantage through economies of scale and pulls higher intellectual life down to the level of the lowest common denominator.[143–145]

Oppressive effects of this process are seen today in direction of extramural funding for universities by the dead hand of peer politics[146,147] within a socially sanctioned technical expert class. Control of psychiatric laboratory research by popularly dictated goals funneled through elite administrations bends authentic inquiry into debased compliance with a collective will.[148,149]

A central government bureaucracy reflecting majority consensus in American politics exerts undue and growing influence over the funding of many psychiatric research areas. An article in the *Archives of General Psychiatry*[150] documents that in 1976, the

National Institute of Mental Health, National Institute of Drug Abuse, and National Institute on Alcoholism and Alcohol Abuse controlled less than half of Federal mental health research support; by 1988, that figure rose to almost two thirds. Moreover, grant allocation tilted toward academic medical recipients; from the 1970s to the late 1980s, the portion of extramural grants awarded to medical schools by the National Institutes of Health increased from one third to over one half. The vast majority of these moneys were distributed through the NIH division of research grants, which exercises tight, highly organized control over routing of funds.[151]

Centralization also increasingly afflicts support of psychiatric research by private philanthropies. It has been observed that those foundations funding psychiatric research are disproportionately large compared to the overall size of surveyed charities.[152]

Not surprisingly, institutions and bureaucracies involved in psychological research with specialized and limited aims often promote funding only in their own restricted areas of interest.[153] Supporters of government funding for the development of specialized psychiatric services tend to be precisely those agencies whose existence is justified and furthered by appropriately dedicated grants.[154] Philanthropic sources also route research funding toward their own parochial areas of concern, while commercial funding of psychoactive drug research is shaped by overt profit motives.[155] Hence, financial compartmentalization increasingly determines the overall subdisciplinary structure of psychiatry. And among these special interests, competition for dominance can be fierce.

Psychiatrists, like everyone else, may feel a desire to dominate.[156] Ruling psychiatric cliques emerge in settings most afflicted with factional competition for funds. Division of labor within institutions thus encourages psychiatric oligarchies.[157-159] So do some professional values of the larger medical community,[160,161] insofar as the modern physician retains his traditional role as an authority figure.[162]

Academic[163] bureaucracies at university medical centers are often low on funds, hierarchically organized, and bound to medical models. It is no wonder, then, that psychiatrists in the employ of such institutions might attempt to improve their own status by treating mental disorders as physical diseases.[164,165]

In America today, biological psychiatry is sliding into financial and administrative control of mental health care. Disturbing tendencies may lurk behind its hunger for medical technology as a means of judging and controlling human behavior. The illusory prospect of infinite malleability in human nature feeds the sense of power that a psychosurgeon or pharmacologist can exercise over other individuals. In the right hands and for the right reasons, of course, brain operations and psychoactive drugs can decrease human suffering. But without constant attention to the diverse motives of those who use them, these and other therapeutic tools can become instruments of control. To whatever extent neuropsychiatry eschews examination of its own psychological origins, potential for abuse exists. Where blind neuropsychiatric technology runs human affairs, the nobler aspirations of psychology may be perverted in its service.

Proponents of biological psychiatry now enjoy new avenues of influence. The efficiency of neurotechnology appeals to popular demands for cost-consciousness in health care. Use of medication benefits the pharmaceutical industry.[166,167] Expert professional witnesses are of use in criminal trials regarding the role of brain damage in the insanity defense of violent behavior.[168–170]

Situations like these have opened up because of the crucial theoretical link between modern normative economics and the neuropsychiatric view of mental pathology. We have been laying groundwork to understand the tie-in, and it can now easily be seen.

A related analysis by the French philosopher Michel Foucault (1926–1984) will be helpful here. Foucault, educated at the École Normale Supérieure and the Sorbonne, earned a doctorate with his book *Madness and Civilization*. He subsequently became head of the philosophy departments at two French universities and produced many writings, including *The Birth of the Clinic* in 1963, on the subject of deviance and power. His fame and authority grew to such an extent during his lifetime that he ultimately replaced Jean-Paul Sartre as France's leading intellectual.[171–173]

Foucault held that every person's boundaries are confined by uncontrollable historical forces which serve the impersonal interests of institutional power. Power operates to expunge from consciousness culturally unacceptable aspects of the self. In a social context, this means that definitions of "normality" require the isolation and disenfranchisement of "abnormal" people.[174,175]

Foucault specifically addressed the ways in which power and normality generate contemporary psychiatric practices. He claimed that madmen were tolerated as an integral part of community life during feudal times, but became segregated in roles as patients after the birth of modern capitalism's work ethic. At that time, Foucault asserted, mental illness became associated with indolence, and its quarantine thus followed as a matter of course.[176–180]

The all-embracing nature of today's market mentality cannot help but lead its norms to act in the coercive manner described by Foucault. Markets not only monopolize broad social agendas but also absorb private desires. They determine the public roles of society's members, yet also distort those fragments of individual selves that define narrow appetites.[181] The internally disruptive impact of interpersonal exchanges in our economic environment assaults the individual through alienated labor so that, in psychoanalytic terms, he "cannot maintain the integrity and wholeness of his experience of himself within his . . . relations with others and is forced to fragment himself to maintain . . . those relations."[182] Thus, modern man has no choice but to throw himself into the collective welter of compulsive work if he wants to think of himself as "normal." Economic symmetry between internal and social imperatives hence damages individual autonomy by deforming it into a workaholic commodity.[183–185]

The autonomous "individual" thereby repressed is simply somatic selfhood, which has been split off by torsional symmetry-breaking from the economic interplay between collective and fragmentary self-identities.[186] Repressed somatic selves constitute individual aspects of human existence that, not fitting into normative economics, must be reduced to "aberrant" objects of diagnosis and collective ostracism.

Neuropsychiatric misconceptions of mental illness therefore stem from and reinforce torsion's fracture of selfhood into economic and somatic subgroups. This happens because if the economic element is normative, then the aberrant component must be somatic. That is the real underlying link between the market mentality and neuropsychiatry.

11

Neuropsychiatry and Psychoanalysis

We have seen that biological psychiatry's vaunted cost-effectiveness is a circular concept. Its very handling of mental health as a material commodity stems from quantitative definitions of efficiency that are influenced by economics.[1–3] These definitions imply a mode of "normal"[4] living that fuels the modern market. They exclude as a "disease" deviation from commercially exploitable behavior.

Fragments of the resulting schism between mental normality and illness thus end up opposing each other in the economic arena. On the stronger side stands commodity-oriented "normality." On the weaker side is the repressed self, labeled as "abnormal." Neuroscience, as a normalizing influence robustly supported by today's commonly held social values, thus has the upper hand.

However, there is a flip side to all this. That other aspect, which can help restore balance to neuropsychiatry, is psychoanalysis, invented by Sigmund Freud.[5]

Freud was born in Schlossergasse, Moravia, on May 6, 1856. He moved with his family four years later to Vienna, where he lived until the Nazis drove him out in 1938. As a child Freud became inspired by the theories of Darwin and by Goethe's essay

"On Nature" to become a medical scientist. He overcame the obstacle of anti-Semitism in medical school and managed to do some basic research in neuroscience under the tutelage of professors Ernst Brucke and Theodore Meynert. As a student Freud also heard Franz Brentano speak.

Finances forced Freud to abandon the laboratory for a clinical career. In 1885, he obtained a grant to study at the Salpêtrière Hospital in Paris. There he worked under the famous neurologist Jean-Martin Charcot and learned about the phenomenon of hysteria.

Freud returned to Vienna the following year, married, and opened a private medical practice. Initially he worked as a neurologist. However, he soon abandoned the neurological approach in many of his cases and instead explored their psychological dimensions. He also withdrew from the academic world and professional societies, which were not friendly to his viewpoint.

Using clinical material obtained in collaboration with a colleague, Josef Breuer, Freud published his first psychoanalytic work, *Studies in Hysteria*, in 1885. Thereafter, Freud parted company with Breuer, developed psychoanalysis on his own, and produced such famous writings as *The Interpretation of Dreams* (1900), *The Psychopathology of Everyday Life* (1904), and *Jokes and Their Relation to the Unconscious* (1905). Eventually, a circle of disciples, including Jung, Abraham, Adler, Reich, Rank, Ferenczi, and Stekel, formed around him. He was invited to speak at Clark University in Massachusetts in 1909; his talk there helped to spark the growth of an international psychoanalytic community that organized learned societies and published professional journals. Meanwhile, Freud pushed forward in his theoretical insights through such books as *The Ego and the Id* (1923). By the time Freud died of cancer in London in 1939, his fame had been secured.[6–10]

Freud's thought was inspired but far from perfect. He has been attacked repeatedly in the era of modern neuropsychiatry for many of his ideas. A number of empirically oriented psychologists are especially put off by the ostensibly subjective nature of his methods. These critics have charged that the clinical "facts" on which Freud claimed to base his theories were obtained as anecdotes with no rigorous controls; resulting psychoanalytic inferences thus allegedly reflected only Freud's power of suggestion over patients in his thrall. Opponents have also indicted Freud for willfully suppressing inconvenient objective findings, autocratic behavior toward colleagues, ineffective treatment techniques, anthropomorphism, circular logic, and overinclusive reasoning. The paradoxical idea of "reaction formation," by which a phenomenon can be explained not only by its apparent motivation but also by an opposite wish, has drawn particular fire.[11-15]

Some of these charges may contain an element of truth. However, it should be noted that Freud sought proof of his ideas not only through intangible psychotherapeutic effects on neuroses and other "treatable" mental disorders. He also looked for independent, objective evidence in similarities between morbidly neurotic behavior and healthy phenomena, such as dreams, jokes, and slips of the tongue.[16]

Nevertheless, crude caricatures of psychoanalysis have helped over the years to give Freud's theory a somewhat worse name than it deserves. Critics have held up reified Freudian maps of abstract mental "regions" specializing in esoteric functions as prime examples of vulgar psychoanalytic monstrosities. The earliest such map was Freud's division of the psyche into conscious, preconscious, and unconscious parts. Later, that model was traded for the concepts of ego, id, and superego.[17] Freud viewed both tripartite[18,19] schemes as mere heuristic devices, but some followers cast them in concrete and thus provided ammunition for opponents.

In an effort to improve the appeal of psychoanalysis to biologically oriented empirical scientists, a tendency to reduce psychoanalytic ideas to neural terms has arisen in some quarters. Many trying to embed Freudian notions in a neuroscientific mold have invoked the ideas of Conwy Lloyd Morgan, John Hughlings Jackson, and Paul MacLean. Their theories, it will be recalled, suggest that mental health depends on a balance between higher cerebral centers and the primitive instinctual structures that they selectively inhibit. A few scientists have thus looked for id-like analogues in limbic brain regions. Others have cited the most up-to-date research on anxiety, a topic of great interest to Freud, and connected it with neural activity in the locus ceruleus of the brainstem.[20,21]

Claims that Freud himself was a mechanistic materialist attempt to justify such reductions. Freud's *Project for a Scientific Psychology* and his early "libido" theory are frequently cited as evidence. The *Project* set an agenda for interpreting mental life as brain phenomena. Libido theory likened the psyche to a "hydraulic" fluid that could either find healthy outlets or dam up under pressure from blocked emotions, leading to neurotic leaks in unhealthy regions of mental life. Libido theory also invoked a "pleasure principle" of psychological tension reduction whose feedback properties tied it to mechanical concepts of homeostasis and cybernetics.[22]

The truth is that all Freud's materialistic ideas originated in early prejudices, which did not last. They were nineteenth-century holdovers that had induced him to begin his medical career in neurology instead of psychiatry and then lost their influence on him.[23] Although Freud did claim to be a materialist early in his career, he really was not as time went on.[24] After he finally recognized the defects of neurological approaches, Freud documented his changed views by writing:

> My therapeutic arsenal [in Vienna of the late 1880s] contained only two weapons, electrotherapy and hypnotism. . . . My knowledge of electrotherapy was derived from W. Erb's textbook, which provided detailed instructions for the treatment of all the symptoms of nervous diseases. Unluckily I was soon driven to see that following these instructions was of no help whatever and that what I had taken for an epitome of exact observations was merely the construction of phantasy. The . . . work of the greatest name in neuropathology had no more relation to reality than some "Egyptian" dream-book, such as is sold

in cheap bookshops. . . . So I put my electrical apparatus aside. . . .[25]

Freud started to recognize that his methods of psychotherapy worked not for simple objective reasons but because of self-reflection, which resisted controlled measurement and hence could not qualify as orthodox neuroscientific evidence.[26] As Rieff has pointed out, Freud generated self-reference through "his willingness to pronounce judgments and draw out the evidence for them from his own life as well as from clinical data."[27] Current psychoanalytic practices still bow to the need for self-reflection. Each professional psychoanalytic trainee must himself be psychoanalyzed. Even after a candidate graduates from an institute, examination of his own inner life continues to play a key role in his effectiveness in treating patients.

Psychoanalysis, like any mental process that self-referently provides a mirror for its own thoughts, acts in a paradoxical manner that transcends orderly logic. Such transcendence, like all mastery of paradox, must be achieved through intentionality.[28,29] Hence, as pointed out by Arnold Cooper of the Payne Whitney Clinic in New York City, psychoanalysis reveals itself as "an attempt to decode . . . meanings" in mental life.[30] Moreover, the semantic content of Freudian investigation goes beyond mere conscious intentionality; it explores unconscious meanings as well.[31–33]

The idea of an intentionally unconscious mental domain is not only self-referent[34]; it is *doubly* self-referent. This becomes apparent when word substitutions are made in the general statement "John Doe is unconscious of a thing." The intentionality of consciousness forces us to include an object, the word "thing," in the sentence. If "I am" replaces "John Doe is" and "my unconsciousness" replaces "a thing," the result is a Freudian assertion that "I am unconscious of my unconsciousness." Two paradoxes inhere in this sentence: that I (the conscious utterer of this sentence) am unconscious and that the object of my unconsciousness is my unconsciousness.

Because of the double paradox intrinsic to unconscious meaning, illogic of a particularly deep kind rules the Freudian mind, whose lowest regions churn with irrational passion and conflict. Reason exerts no influence down in its recesses; contradictory desires and beliefs coexist through the doubly illogical mental mode known as "primary process thinking."

Freud first gained access to this unconscious, two-layered realm of unreason by considering the content of dreams, amplified through a form of psychological exploration known as "free association."[35] He asked his patients to recount their experiences during sleep and then let their minds wander, uncensored, to other thoughts spurred by dream recollections.

Through this method, he concluded that reported dreams were "overdetermined" by unconscious wishes that were many times more frangibly abundant than events in the dreams themselves. Unconscious contradictions, which the conscious reasoning abilities of his patients could not reconcile, fused into terse but distorted dream symbols and additional nonsensical items instead of straightforward, logical assertions. They were thus "condensed" into consciousness during the course of dream expression. A related example of such fusion is compromise formation, an unconscious defense that both expresses and disguises forbidden desires.[36]

All such condensed phenomena constituted a first tier of irrationality, which Freud was able to contact by free-associative methods. The second tier involved "transference," the irrational attachment that a patient often forms with his psychotherapist. Some of Freud's successors attempted to handle this phenomenon through the device of doubly self-referent empathic interplay between patient and therapist. For these post-Freudians, psychotherapeutic empathy functioned not as an impersonal technical ploy but as a surrogate for fungible self-reflection. In such a mirrorlike process, the therapist endeavored to assume his patient's subjective viewpoint. It was hoped that the patient's reaction to his therapist as an inquiring, coequal partner and conduit to self-exploration would thus itself feed back through the therapist's understanding. The immediacy of resulting insights might hence reflect a patient's honest, committed contact with his own balanced selfhood and therefore tap into his natural ability to heal himself as a whole organism.[37]

The empathic approach was developed by a number of innovative psychotherapists. Chief among them were Harry Stack Sullivan (1892–1949) and Carl Jung (1875–1961).

Sullivan was born in Norwich, New York. He overcame great difficulties on the path toward his achievements in psychoanalysis. Sullivan suffered persecution as a Roman Catholic in a small town during his childhood. He received spotty formal education, spending only one year in college and graduating from a medical school that he himself called "a diploma mill." Nonetheless, he learned about psychoanalysis from a friend, Clara Thompson, and earned specialty certification through psychiatric work with the armed forces. Sullivan's thought added critical interpersonal perspectives, inspired by discussions with the anthropologist Edward Sapir, to Freud's ideas.[38,39]

Jung came from a family of Swiss clergymen and physicians. As a student, he became interested in both paleontology and comparative religion, a dichotomy that carried over into his mature thought. It led him toward the specialty of psychiatry after he had attended medical school in Basel and read the introduction to a well-known textbook on psychopathology. He began his career as an assistant under Eugen Bleuler in the Burgholzli Mental Hospital. Jung invented a diagnostic word-association test at Burgholzli and went on to develop an interest in the writings of Freud, whom he met a few years later and whose circle he joined. Jung became the first president of the International Psychoanalytic Association and edited its *Jahrbuch*. However, disagreements over theoretical concepts led to a split with Freud in 1912. Thereafter, Jung worked alone to develop his own psychotherapeutic approach. He called his conceptual framework "analytical psychology" and based it on anthropological evidence for the collective nature of unconscious symbolism. Jung's thought emphasized the "synchronous" link between internal and other-directed mental life. His psychology stipulated that therapy must involve mutuality, in which both the doctor and the patient invest their inner and outer being.[40-43]

Though Freud's concept of mutual interchange in his relationships with patients was less developed than the empathic perspectives of Sullivan and Jung, his interest in open interdisciplinary dialogue ranged widely. Freud's sources for psychoanalysis were eclectic: They subsumed, for example, concepts from nineteenth-century physics as well as characters from Sophocles' plays.[44] His developmental understanding of psychiatric symptoms included multiple factors,[45] and his views about the origin of anxiety derived from both evolutionary theory and introspective psychology.[46]

Eclecticism spilled over into the work of Freud's disciples. This included not only the thought of Sullivan and Jung but also Alfred Adler's individual psychology, Karen Horney's holistic approach, and Sandor Ferenczi's active therapy. Related schools emerged from such sources as linguistics, anthropology, and Gestalt psychology. The practice of psychotherapy attracted many gifted adherents, among whom continual debate and intellectual ferment had a synergistic, productive impact.[47-50]

Psychoanalytic therapists have not held a monopoly on empathic interchange or eclectic theories. Another great master of psychological and intellectual breadth was William James (1842–1910). James was born in New York City to a wealthy and cultured family, with whom he traveled extensively during childhood. His father, Henry James, Sr., was a well-known theologian, and his brother, Henry, Jr., became a respected novelist. Through a wide variety of experiences facilitated by his family fortune, James became educated in many fields. He studied painting, spoke several languages fluently, explored the jungles of Brazil, and earned a Harvard medical degree. At the age of 30, James accepted a faculty appointment in physiology at Harvard, later moving into the psychology and philosophy departments. In 1878, he married and began a 12-year-writing project, culminating in his book *Principles of Psychology* in 1890. A second masterwork,

The Varieties of Religious Experience, was published in 1902 and a third, *Pragmatism*, in 1907.

In all these writings, a highly pluralistic outlook expanding the thought of pragmatist Charles S. Peirce informed James's discussions of the human mind. His eclectic fluidity could also be appreciated in his contacts with such diverse luminaries as Emerson, Freud, Wundt, Mach, and Russell and by contrasting his religious writings with his establishment of an experimental psychology laboratory at Harvard in 1875. James was almost alone among his nineteenth-century American peers in retaining a desire to reconcile "objective" biological considerations and the complexity of subjective experience. His singular empathic bent also led him to investigate alien conscious experiences such as psychic, supranormal, and pathological mental states.[51-57]

Still other eclectic individuals, eager for sympathetic interchange with viewpoints contrary to their own, have operated in fields related to psychology. Exchanges between the European and Oriental religious concepts of mind trace their history from Alexander the Great's contact with India in 325 BC, through Jones's discovery of links between Sanskrit and European languages and Schopenhauer's Germanic embrace of Eastern religion, and into more recent Western interest in meditative explorations of consciousness. Synergy has also informed some purely European philosophy. Wittgenstein's thought married positivism and existentialism. Logic mixed with intentionality formed a new literary discipline called critical hermeneutics.[58] Metaeconomists like Weber, Veblen, and the Frankfurt School achieved their insights because they reached out to more than one discipline.[59]

In areas of science related to sociobiology, the concept of the gene as a chainlike molecule took form historically in the musings not only of biologists but also of quantum scientists like Erwin Schrödinger and Max Delbruck.[60] During the 1930s, the physicist Niels Bohr had suggested that the principles of atomic physics might be relevant to biological research. Delbruck and Schrödinger then formulated more specific hypotheses about the chemical nature of the gene. Data from electron microscopy, chemical analyses, and x-ray crystallography obtained by Linus Pauling, Maurice Wilkins, and Rosalind Franklin then allowed Francis Crick and James Watson to crack the genetic code. Among all these people, Crick, Wilkins, Bohr, Delbruck, Schrödinger, and others had training as physicists under their belts.[61]

Schrödinger himself wrote that

> when examining what are called . . . *different* views of the same object . . . one . . . should, instead of stressing the *contradictions* between them, . . . aim at combining these different aspects into one total picture.[62]

Intellectual growth has always demanded interchange among seemingly opposing viewpoints. As John Stuart Mill wrote:

> It is hardly possible to overrate the value . . . of placing human beings in contact with . . . modes of thought and action unlike those with which they are familiar. . . . Such communication has always been . . . one of the primary sources of [authentic] progress.[63]

Only conceptual synergy through interdisciplinary dialogue will allow the inquiring agent to turn his apparently limited perspective inside-out and conduct meaningful conversations with himself in the same kind of critical language that he uses in talking to others. Only thus will he be able to merge social objects with his own subjectivity in order to generate new self-concepts from honest debate.[64,65] The inquiring agent must gain "the ability to see things as others do" in order to perceive "the pluralism of the world."[66] In this way, the self will benefit from opportunities for interactive discovery.

Psychology more than any other field of study needs interdisciplinary dialogue and empathic insight into alien subjective viewpoints. The doubly self-referent nature of unconscious intentionality requires it; intentionally barren paradigms alone will not satisfy the demand. Even as famous a researcher as Francois Jacob has stated that his own kind of "hard" science is "diluted out in the study of man, . . . one approach among others."[67]

Prospective psychiatrists might enrich the present, biologically restricted content of their chosen field through greater breadth of learning both during and after training. Premedical candidates, who feed the pool of future research psychiatrists, might try to escape the narrowing influence of specialized technical training[68] through course work in quantum or relativity theories, which hone abilities to think in new and nonmechanical ways. Medical school admission committees might also demand a solid background in nonscientific subjects such as anthropology, history, and philosophy. They might consider accepting more students who have journeyed beyond the dryness of numerical pseudotruth into the range and depth of subjective understanding offered by literary works like *Hamlet*, *The Book of Job*, and *Crime and Punishment*.

Desirable role models offered to students might include Sigmund Freud or William James. The flexibility demonstrated by these intellectual adventurers enhanced psychiatry's understanding in the past. Disciplined eclecticism like theirs today might help to mend the asymmetries of reduced interdisciplinary dialogue fostered by neurobiological myopia. Opposing definitions of disease and of treatment efficacy integrated in the right spirit would thereby enhance psychiatry. Young trainees might thus look forward to a new psychiatric world that represents an open, multidisciplinary "democracy of the intellect,"[69] encompassing all the various camps relevant to psychiatry.

However, eclectic flexibility involves risk[70] that requires seeing beyond neuropsychiatry's short-term financial appeal. A risky venture like psychology or psychiatry guarantees no particular result and always leaves a chance of failure, but without ongoing risk there would exist no possibility for growth and success.[71] James knew this, and so did Freud. Psychoanalysis defies technical standards of exact scientific proof; the subjectivity of Freudian treatment methods bestow on therapeutic effects an inconsistency that eludes empirical cost-benefit analysis.[72,73] The protean aspects of psychoanalytic thought, moreover, have outlived Freud and impelled evolution of his methods in the hands of disciples and students into unanticipated forms that its author might barely recognize. As the years have passed since Freud's death and the spectrum of patients has changed, his brand of psychotherapy has mutated accordingly, with an increase in the importance of risk and empathy. Freud's least empathic trademark, the couch, has disappeared in many consultation rooms.[74,75]

The existentialist philosophers have had a large influence on post-Freudian psychotherapy. The most important of these thinkers was Søren Kierkegaard (1813–1855), a native of Copenhagen whose life was tinged with tragedy. He had a malformed spine, his parents and five of his six siblings died by the time he reached early adulthood, and his one love affair ended unhappily. Although Kierkegaard showed a smiling demeanor to others, he remained privately somber much of the time. He studied theology at the University of Copenhagen and then opted for the life of an isolated intellectual, criticizing the rationalistic hypocrisy that afflicted his society and church. His writings included *Either-Or*, *Fear and Trembling*, *The Sickness unto Death*, and *The Concept of Dread*. He is said to have criticized his own books in anonymous reviews.[76–78] Kierkegaard emphasized the importance of flexibility and freedom in choosing modes of autoinvention. He argued forcefully that meaningful commitment to courageous leaps with the expansive potential for diverse outcomes is crucial in determining the means by which the creative efforts of psychology direct self-understanding.[79–82]

These ideas were taken up by psychiatrists like Victor Frankl, R. D. Laing, and especially Karl Jaspers (1883–1969). Jaspers was born in Oldenburg, Germany. He worked at first as a psychiatrist at the University of Heidelberg, where he came to embrace the ideas of Max Weber and oppose the influence of Kraepelin's methodological rigor. In 1913, he published the book *General Psychopathology*, which presented his view of an empathic, existentially oriented psychiatry. In 1916, he moved to Heidelberg's philosophy department, and he joined the faculty of the University of Basel in Switzerland in 1948.[83]

Jaspers himself was a paragon of existential courage. At great personal risk, he opposed Nazi practices based on materialistic racial theories and became an influential voice in the rebuilding of Heidelberg's academic infrastructure after 1945. His bravery showed how existentialist values can ennoble psychiatry in particular and life in general.

The haziness of existential risk, however, is difficult for those seeking absolute "scientific" proof to tolerate. Switching among mutually exclusive paradigms creates cognitive dissonance.[84] Hence, theoretical ambiguity unnerves many scientific psychologists hostile to the existential aspect of psychoanalytic thought. Some may experience outright dread or anxiety.

Anxiety is disorganizing, disorienting, and painful,[85,86] yet it is also a universal and recurrent feature of human life.[87] Ernest Becker, Pulitzer Prize–winning author of *The Denial of Death*, points out that man in general "is an ambiguous creature . . . [who] can never [really] banish anxiety."[88] Moreover, the existential anxiety associated with risk, though unpleasant, is in fact far from pathological. On the contrary, tolerance of anxiety may be a sign of emotional health and existential awareness.[89] Constructive anxiety may herald spontaneous and autonomous action,[90] which depends on our proclivity for diffuse, objectless curiosity, uncoupled from any drive for predictable outcomes of our actions.[91,92] Only through open-ended exploration can potentially constructive risk-taking in the study of mental life actually help us to navigate unpredictable turns in the labyrinth of the measurable world.

Man, by facing rather than denying his most diffuse fears, can muster the courage to use existential ambivalence as a springboard for growth into new realms of thought. He can exploit anxiety as an ongoing "school" that opens up truth through firsthand subjective engagement with everyday risk. Such a path can allow us to move on toward authentic autonomy.[93] Ortega y Gasset described this eloquently:

> The man with the clear head is the man who . . . looks life in the face, realizes that everything in it is problematic,

and feels himself lost. And this is the simple truth, that to live is to feel oneself lost—he who accepts it has already begun to find himself, to be on firm ground. Instinctively, as do the shipwrecked, he will look round for something to which to cling, and that tragic, ruthless glance, absolutely sincere, because of this question of his salvation, will cause him to bring order into the chaos of his life. These are the only genuine ideas: the ideas of the shipwrecked. All the rest is rhetoric, posturing, farce.[94]

Freud's purposeful ambiguity, which has spawned anxiety among some critics, provides elbow room in case of "shipwrecks." It has left us space for possible revisions in Freud's theories on the basis of changes that he anticipated in physical science. Freud advised fellow psychoanalysts of his time to be "content with fragmentary pieces of knowledge and with basic hypotheses lacking in preciseness" because he looked forward to a future "emergence of more extensive and deeper-reaching natural laws" to which his inheritors should be "ready to submit"[95] in the interest of greater self-consciousness.

Becker explains that man's one great "penalty" for self-consciousness is anxiety, because true self-awareness includes "knowledge of one's own death."[96] Freud's counterintuitive idea of Thanatos, his "death instinct,"[97] addresses the technician's dread of ambiguity in psychoanalysis. It accounts for the fact that the "ritualized activity" of at least some psychiatrists operating in the biological tradition serves to shield the clinician from the "anxiety of his or her own human condition by emphasizing the difference, and the distance, between physician and patient." That difference puts up a wall between "the physician as the one who has the specialized esoteric knowledge and the patient as the one who has the [potentially lethal] disease."[98]

Freud initially invoked Thanatos to explain why shell-shocked World War I veterans obsessively relived the emotional traumas of battle. He termed this tendency "repetition compulsion" and began to flirt with the idea that some human actions are motivated by irreducible unconscious urges for pain and self-dissolution. Phillip Rieff recounts that later,[99] in Freud's mature thought, death itself became

> more than a bodily event; . . . [it became unconsciously] willed. This is the road . . . [Freud] took with the "death instinct," first enunciated in *Beyond the Pleasure Principle* (1920). In 1938, a year before he died of cancer, he suspected that we die not merely of disease, but of the death-wish. . . ; ageless Thanatos asserts itself "until it at length succeeds in doing the individual to death."[100]

Freud meant Thanatos to operate in opposition to his earlier, restricted concept of Eros, a hedonic, "tension-reducing" hunger for pleasure. He thus postulated the intrapsychic coexistence of erotic and destructive instincts locked in conflict with each other.[101] In this sense, Freud internalized the existential concept of man as a "union of opposites."[102] He believed that people must constantly rise to the challenge of mediating between their own intrinsic erotic and self-destructive wishes.

The intuited risk of a fatal outcome in the conflict between Eros and Thanatos generates anxiety. Dread signals an impending volitional gamble through an adventurous leap that, with terrifying uncertainty, may either promote or injure self-integrity. The resulting existential dilemma therefore is neither abstract, in the manner of mathematical absurdities like those concocted by Russell and Gödel, nor merely metaphysical, in the manner of puzzles posed by Descartes, nor even methodological, like the *modus tollens* aspects of Popperian science. It is instead concrete and ever-present in a terrible and immediate sense. At any time our own most seductive impulses may reduce us to "food for worms," and we know it.[103]

Freud's concept of a war between Eros and Thanatos relates psychoanalysis to the alienated somatic self of modern economic life. It implies that the pleasure-seeking goals of mass consumption hide latent drives toward bodily death. This insight gives us a liberating "way forward"[104] from the crass delusions of normative ideology that now imprison psychiatry.[105] Freudian aims transcend tensions that lead "normal" technical science,[106] connected with commerce and utility, to deny or ignore Thanatos and hence allow destructive appetites to run wild.

Free psychoanalytic self-scrutiny involving Thanatos may help neuroscientists see their somatic orientation in a historical and cultural context. A number of psychoanalytic thinkers have likened human history itself to pathological phenomena, through which primordially repressed, unconscious content resurfaces in ever-steeper death-oriented cycles of self-alienated repetition compulsion. The process leads us from the mythical simplicity of our primeval ancestors to an illusion of human progress that in truth reflects only historical needs of the regressive social stages in which human awareness has been buried. In this scheme we first encounter the image of an erotic[107] phase of history, organizing humans into families and archaic agricultural communities tied to the cycles of fertility rites. Later we see more agonistic[108] issues of money and debt propel the compulsive technical efficiency of commerce and industry. Finally we come upon our own anonymous time, obsessed with the atomizing issues of consumption[109] and quantitative pseudoidentity that obscure psychological reality.[110–116]

Psychoanalysis can use this kind of understanding to infuse neuroscience with a new, intentionally self-choosing power.[117] Psychoanalytic methods can separate and plumb the myriad unconscious historical meanings[118] underlying the facade of formal symbolic[119] architectures that represent today's research paradigms in neurobiology. Toward this end, psychoanalytic inquiry tells us that we need no longer hide from the subjectivity latent beneath "objective" science, but should instead fathom and resolve it.[120]

Elements of psychoanalytic exploration may even act to inform a scientist's deliberate selections of particular neural relationships and architectures for different research subjects; it can prevent this voluntary choice from collapsing into a narrow, deadening search for definitive brain "mechanisms." Volkow and Tancredi have pointed out that "differences among . . . strategies used to process a given stimulus may lead to differences in the patterns of [brain] activation in response to the stimulus." For example, subjects attempting to remember auditory tones using an analytical approach activate the left half of the brain, while those employing a nonanalytical style utilize the right. The particular neural substrate that comes into play depends on a choice between different mnemonic strategies. As long as the choosing agent himself remains wary of the death instinct's potential role in his selection, conceiving mental life as a menu offering different neural alternatives can lose at least some of its life-denying power.[121]

Consciousness of self-destructive urges can expand our ability to cope with the many possible corrupting demands of neuropsychiatric progress. This expansion can create a payoff in the pace and direction of future scientific growth. Psychoanalytic recall, through a reacquaintance with the most primitive and undifferentiated sources of our human potential, can rejuvenate our range of neurobiological options.[122–124] It can give us flexible access to alternative modes of consciousness across the continua of phylogeny, ranging from simple cell systems to complex states of human brain arousal.[125] It can stretch across the entire span of cerebral ontogeny,[126] from infancy to death itself. Psychoanalytic inquiry can thereby force the empirically given falsity of all our somatic guises and brain states,[127,128] appearing to succeed each other in time, into self-corrective[129] confrontation with their own mortal limits.

In this way, psychoanalysis can interact synergistically with neuroscience.[130] The two approaches, each with its own viewpoints, strengths, and weaknesses,[131] can help one another blossom. Their roles in this synergy, however, must remain distinct. Psychoanalytic concepts, with their double layer of self-reference and intentionality, can never reduce to the mechanistic materialism of biology. Instead, neuroscience stands in relation to psychoanalysis as what Kandel and Wilson have called an "antidiscipline." Freudian intentionality can pose meaningful questions and hypotheses that direct neuroscientific inquiry; neurobiology, armed with new research tools, can try to separate fact from fiction among psychoanalytic speculations.[132] Neuroscience hence may help put alternative forms of psychoanalytic theory into empirically testable form[133] and thereby affect views on psychoanalytically relevant issues like childhood development.[134]

The studies of Hubel, Wiesel, Harlow, and others concerning the psychobiology of infant growth are already performing this kind of service; they have made many psychoanalysts more open in their work to information other than patients' anecdotes, useful as those may be.[135,136] Hubel and Wiesel have shown specifically that critical periods of synaptic change exist in cats during their first months of life. Only within these intervals are certain junctions between cells still unformed and subject to molding by outside forces for better or worse. Harry Harlow's work has revealed critical periods, like those of young synapses, in the gross behavior of monkeys. He observed that infant animals without the soft touch of a mother or some suitable substitute during important phases of their infancies become mentally disturbed. All these data have invited inferences about the interplay among transmitters, early psychological trauma, and human emotional derangement.[137]

The psychiatrist's conscious awareness of unconscious intentionality can help direct multidisciplinary approaches to clinical management.[138] There is evidence that psychoanalytically informed psychotherapy integrated with medication and other biologically based treatments often improves the recovery of psychiatric patients. For severe personality disorders and some instances of depression, an exploratory psychotherapeutic component may be absolutely required.[139–141] Schizophrenia also fares best when tactful, empathic support of a patient and his family undergirds pharmacotherapy.[142–145]

In many instances, psychiatric symptoms with apparent biological causes may harbor deep meaning for an individual patient.[146] For example, triggers for phobias, obsessive–compulsive behavior, and panic attacks may involve psychologically significant events, like enraging situations or the threatened loss of a loved one, that set known physiological mechanisms in motion. Psychoanalytic exploration can uncover such triggers and help at least some patients deal with them. Medication may function only to block the disorganizing effects of anxiety and thus pull these patients together in order to begin insight-oriented work.[147–151]

Pharmacotherapy and inpatient confinement per se have meanings to patients that may affect compliance with and response to biological treatments.[152] As Anna Spielvogel, director of residency training at San Francisco General Hospital, has stated, "If we don't understand our patients, we are not going to get them to take their medication."[153] Unless a psychiatrist understands the emotional consequences of hospital admission, he or she may also make poor use of that option. Psychoanalytic theory can assist in these matters.

Psychotherapeutic maneuvers with subjective meaning may even alter the brain all by themselves.[154] Glenn Gabbard of the Menninger Memorial Hospital points out that "psychological interventions in a treatment context may have a profound impact on neurophysiology."[155] Psychotherapy produces the same brain changes as pharmacotherapy in PET scans of obsessive–compulsive patients,[156] who often respond to placebo medication.[157]

ᐠᐤ   ᐠᐤ   ᐠᐤ

Psychoanalysis continues to attract attention even in the "Decade of the Brain" because it represents a helpful addition to the understanding of mental life in two different ways. First, Freud's legacy, like that of Husserl, provides a continuum of concepts that extends naturally, without additional constructs, from health into states that might be regarded as pathological. This reflects respect for "delusional" or otherwise "morbid" mental contents as legitimate objects of study. It mandates the psychiatrist to grant his patients' fantasies a complementary place alongside the hard-headed "realism" of empirical science.[158-161]

Second, the double-tiered intentionality of psychoanalysis provides an existential route not only to diagnosis but also to treatment.[162] Herein, according to one analyst, lies a "chance for real change" through "the vehicle of the [meaningful] quest."[163] Psychoanalysis can thus help us become autonomous decision-makers and free us from normative, culture-bound delusions. The broken symmetry that isolates somatic self-identity[164] in a deadening neuroscientific prison may thereby heal.[165,166]

Psychiatry might then bloom into a truly coherent art with a coordinated understanding of its own overall structure and therapeutic possibilities. Such synoptic self-definition is the goal that students of mental life have sought since the days of ancient Greek philosophy. Inquiring spirits like Pythagoras, Descartes, Spinoza, Brentano, Husserl, and Freud all struggled in different ways to comprehend wide-ranging aspects of the psyche. Pythagoras addressed both numerical and mystical features of thought. Descartes invented the notion of ontological dualism. Spinoza portrayed matter and mind as divergent views of the same underlying reality. Brentano took the mental sciences beyond formal syntax into the realm of intentional meaning. Husserl broadened legitimate psychological discourse to include objects of the imagination. Freud reached down into the soul's core, elaborated two separate tiers of hidden self-reference, applied them to the dual tasks of diagnosis and treatment, and in so doing raised the death instinct to a level of conscious awareness.

Descartes, Brentano, Freud, and the other great philosophers of mind not only synthesized existing knowledge but also broke new ground. None of them could have worked effectively without venturing beyond hallowed conventions to create new viewpoints. In similar fashion, we ourselves may build on the bold achievements of past giants only by contributing our own innovations. The next step on our road to self-knowledge must marshall today's intellectual tools in order to transcend the comfortable old ideas of Thomas Hobbes, expand the perspectives of Baruch Spinoza, balance the insights of Edmund Husserl, and refine the intuitions of Sigmund Freud.

As psychiatry approaches the twenty-first century, its leaders and practitioners must not neglect emerging concepts of meta-mathematics or theories at the cutting edge of post-Newtonian physics. These ideas, either directly or through heuristic analogies, can move us beyond a disjointed picture of the mind. They may allow us to see different traditional approaches to the psyche as related offspring of a more fundamental symmetry principle. Humanity cannot help but benefit from such a unified vision.

Notes

Chapter 1

1. Gerard Piel *et al.*, eds., *The Brain* (San Francisco: W. H. Freeman, 1979), p. 141.
2. Ibid.
3. Nancy Andreasen, *The Broken Brain* (New York: Harper & Row, 1984), p. 152.
4. Eric Kandel, "Psychotherapy and the Single Synapse," *New England Journal of Medicine* 301:19 (8 Nov 1979), p. 1028.
5. Ibid., pp. 1028–1029.
6. Ibid.
7. Andreasen, *The Broken Brain*, pp. 1–2, 37, 141–142, 144–145.
8. Ming T. Tsuang, Stephen V. Faraone, and Max Day, "Schizophrenic Disorders," in *The New Harvard Guide to Psychiatry*, ed. Armand Nicholi (Cambridge: Bellknap Press, 1988), p. 259.
9. Peter McGuffin, "Mental Illness," in *The Oxford Companion to the Mind*, ed. Richard Gregory (Oxford: Oxford University Press, 1987), p. 473.
10. Andreasen, *The Broken Brain*, pp. 36, 63, 53.
11. Harvard Medical School, Department of Continuing Education, *Psychiatry, a Comprehensive Review and Update*, syllabus for course given 6–11 March 1989, p. 71.

12. David Tomb, *Psychiatry for the House Officer* (Baltimore: Williams and Wilkins, 1988), p. 66.
13. Ibid., pp. 66, 69–71.
14. Kenneth Tardiff, "The Current State of Psychiatry in the Treatment of Violent Patients," *Archives of General Psychiatry* 49 (June 1992), pp. 493–495.
15. Tomb, p. 136.
16. "Hippocrates" (no author given), in Gregory, ed., *The Oxford Companion*, p. 312.
17. "Galen (Claudius Galenus)" (no author given), Ibid., p. 281.
18. J. O. Thorne, ed., *Chambers's Biographical Dictionary* (New York: St. Martin's Press, 1962), p. 509.
19. Hippocrates, "The Physiological Bases of Experience," in *Body, Mind, and Death*, ed. Anthony Flew (New York: Macmillan, 1964), pp. 32–33.
20. L. S. Hearnshaw, *The Shaping of Modern Psychology* (London: Routledge, 1987), pp. 151–152.
21. Harold Kaplan and Benjamin Sadock, *Synopsis of Psychiatry* (Baltimore: Williams and Wilkins, 1988), pp. 1–2.
22. Vieda Skultans, "Insanity, Early Theories," in *The Oxford Companion*, p. 372.
23. Jean-Pierre Changeux, *Neuronal Man* (Oxford: Oxford University Press, 1985), p. 11.
24. Kaplan and Sadock, pp. 2, 4.
25. Ibid., p. 7.
26. Thorne, ed., p. 95.
27. Raymond Adams and Maurice Victor, *Principles of Neurology* (New York: McGraw-Hill, 1977), p. 642.
28. W. A. Lishman, *Organic Psychiatry* (Oxford: Blackwell, 1987), pp. 281–282.
29. John Walton, revising author, *Brain's Diseases of the Nervous System* (Oxford: Oxford University Press, 1977), p. 454.
30. Adams and Victor, p. 642.
31. Daniel X. Freedman, "The Search: Body, Mind, and Human Purpose," *American Journal of Psychiatry* 149:7 (July 1992), p. 861.

32. Christian Herriman, "Neurosyphilis," in *Merritt's Textbook of Neurology*, ed. Lewis Rowland (Philadelphia: Lea and Febiger, 1984), p. 123.
33. Kaplan and Sadock, p. 10.
34. Thorne, ed., p. 1342.
35. Walton, p. 468.
36. These developments were in line with the then ascendant germ theory of disease causation, a view promoted by the perfection of the microscope in the nineteenth century and by the work of Louis Pasteur and Robert Koch [Fritjof Capra, *The Turning Point* (New York: Bantam, 1982), pp. 110–111, 127–129].
37. Freedman, pp. 861–862.
38. Andreasen, *The Broken Brain*, p. 14.
39. David Gorman and Jurgen Unutzer, "Brodmann's 'Missing' Numbers," *Neurology* 43 (January 1993), pp. 226–227.
40. Jonathan Winson, *Brain and Psyche* (Garden City: Doubleday, 1985), p. 63.
41. O. L. Zangwill, "Kraepelin, Emil," in Gregory, ed., *The Oxford Companion*, p. 414.
42. Phillip N. Johnson-Laird, *The Computer and the Mind* (Cambridge: Harvard University Press, 1988), pp. 20–21.
43. Kaplan and Saddock, pp. 147–149.
44. James Schellenberg, *Masters of Social Psychology* (New York: Oxford University Press, 1978), p. 63.
45. The search for biological treatment paradigms in psychiatry grew from the germ theory's success in promoting vaccines and antibiotics active against infectious diseases. These techniques, along with other new modalities like insulin treatment for diabetes, encouraged the idea of biological and chemical therapies to deal with mental symptoms (Capra, pp. 111, 131–132).
46. Pragmatic considerations have always been a spur for developing biological methods of treating abnormal behavior. The ancients furnished precedents in their attempts to cure emotional problems by "direct" physical means. The Greek Hip-

pocrates tried to treat hysteria by luring supposedly errant wombs back to their proper anatomical site, using fragrances applied to the vagina. Some physicians, following theories of the Roman Galen, handled their patients' behavioral quirks by removing excess bodily "humors"; blood-letting was the most common example of such a practice (Andreasen, *The Broken Brain*, p. 143).

47. Kaplan and Sadock, p. 528.
48. Andreasen, *The Broken Brain*, pp. 119, 214–215.
49. Kaplan and Sadock, p. 531.
50. Ibid., pp. 528–529, 531.
51. Andreasen, *The Broken Brain*, p. 198.
52. Ross Baldessarini and Jonathan O. Cole, "Chemotherapy," in Nicholi, ed., *The New Harvard Guide*, p. 499.
53. Andreasen, *The Broken Brain*, pp. 191–192.
54. Ibid., pp. 192–193.
55. Baldessarini and Cole, p. 483.
56. Andreasen, *The Broken Brain*, pp. 194–195.
57. Baldessarini and Cole, pp. 507–508.
58. Winson, pp. 194–195.
59. Baldessarini and Cole, pp. 521–523.
60. Tomb, pp. 77, 87–88, 208–210.
61. Andreasen, *The Broken Brain*, p. 193.
62. Ibid., p. 31.
63. Stuart C. Yudofsky and Robert E. Hales, "The Reemergence of Neuropsychiatry: Definition and Direction," *Journal of Neuropsychiatry* 1:1 (Winter 1989), p. 3.
64. Andreasen, *The Broken Brain*, pp. 19, 149–150.

Chapter 2

1. Yudofsky and Hales, "The Reemergence of Neuropsychiatry," p. 4.
2. Andreasen, *The Broken Brain*, pp. 108, 172–173, 176.
3. Nancy Andreasen, Gregg Cohen, Greg Harris, Ted Cizaldo,

Jussi Parkkinen, Karim Rezai, and Victor Swayze, "Image Processing for the Study of Brain Structure and Function: Problems and Programs," *Journal of Neuropsychiatry* 4:2 (Spring, 1992), pp. 125–133.

4. Robert Hendren and Janet Hodde-Vargas, "Neuroimaging in Schizophrenia," *Psychiatric Times* (September 1992), pp. 17–18.

5. Jeffrey Coffman, "Computed Tomography in Psychiatry," in *Brain Imaging: Applications in Psychiatry*, ed. Nancy Andreasen (Washington D.C.: American Psychiatric Press, 1989), pp. 1–3.

6. Nancy Andreasen, "Nuclear Magnetic Resonance Imaging," in Andreasen, ed., *Brain Imaging*, p. 67.

7. Edward Edelson, "Scanning the Body Magnetic," *Science 83* (July–August 1983), pp. 60–65.

8. Michael Devous, "Imaging Brain Function by Single-Photon Emission Computer Tomograph," in Andreasen, ed., *Brain Imaging*, pp. 148–150.

9. Henry Holcomb, Jonathan Links, Caroline Smith, and Dean Wong, "Positron Emission Tomography: Measuring the Metabolic and Neurochemical Characteristics of the Living Human Nervous System," in Andreasen, ed., *Brain Imaging*, pp. 235–236.

10. Sandra Blakeslee, "Scanner Pinpoints Site of Thought as Brain Sees or Speaks," *New York Times* (1 June 1993), pp. C1, C3.

11. Gina Kolata, "Improved Scanner Watches the Brain As It Thinks," *New York Times* (14 July 1992), pp. C1, C6.

12. Nora D. Volkow and Laurence R. Tancredi, "Biological Correlates of Mental Activity Studied With PET," *American Journal of Psychiatry* 148:4 (April 1991), pp. 439–440, 442.

13. Andreasen, *The Broken Brain*, pp. 166–171, 226.

14. Hendren and Hodde-Vargas, pp. 19–20.

15. Tomb, *Psychiatry for the House Officer*, p. 25.

16. Andreasen, *The Broken Brain*, p. 178.

17. Andreasen *et al.*, "Image Processing," pp. 125–133.

18. Ruben Gur, Roland Erwin, and Raquel Gur, "Neurobehavioral

Probes, for Physiologic Neuroimaging Studies," *Archives of General Psychiatry* 49 (May 1992), pp. 409–414.

19. Hendren and Hodde-Vargas, pp. 18–20.

20. Robert Innis, "Neuroreceptor Imaging with SPECT," *Journal of Clinical Psychiatry* 53:11 (November 1992 supplement), pp. 29–34.

21. John Lauerman, "Windows on the Brain: Functional Brain Imaging Techniques Add Objective Scale to Psychiatric Evaluation and Treatment," *Psychiatric Times* (February 1993), pp. 16–17.

22. Donald Mender, notes for lecture on CT, MRI and PET scanning in psychiatry given in 1988 at St. John's Episcopal Hospital, Smithtown, New York.

23. Marc Schuckit, "An Introduction and Overview to Clinical Applications of Neuro SPECT in Psychiatry," *Journal of Clinical Psychiatry* 53:11 (November 1992 supplement), pp. 3–6.

24. Ronald Van Heertum, "Brain SPECT Imaging and Psychiatry," *Journal of Clinical Psychiatry* 53:11 (November 1992 supplement), pp. 7–12.

25. Nora Volkow and Laurence Tancredi, "Current and Future Applications of SPECT in Clinical Psychiatry," *Journal of Clinical Psychiatry* 53:11 (November 1992 supplement), pp. 26–28.

26. Scott Woods, "Regional Cerebral Blood Flow Imaging with SPECT in Psychiatric Disease: Focus on Schizophrenia, Anxiety Disorders, and Substance Abuse," *Journal of Clinical Psychiatry* 53:11 (November 1992 supplement), pp. 20–25.

27. Blakeslee, "Scanner," pp. C–1, C–3.

28. Kolata, pp. C1, C6.

29. Volkow and Tancredi, "Biological Correlates," pp. 439–440, 442.

30. Andreasen, *The Broken Brain*, pp. 28, 120–121, 194, 225, 238.

31. Juan M. De Lecuona, K. Sunny Joseph, Naveed Iqbal, and Gregory Asis, "Dopamine Hypothesis of Schizophrenia Revisited," *Psychiatric Annals* 23:4 (April 1993), pp. 179–185.

32. Tomb, pp. 25–26.

33. Winson, p. 238.
34. Andreasen, *The Broken Brain*, pp. 233–234.
35. Tomb, pp. 42–43, 45–46.
36. Andreasen, *The Broken Brain*, pp. 181–182, 234.
37. Burr Eichelman, "Aggressive Behavior: From Laboratory to Clinic," *Archives of General Psychiatry* 49 (June 1992), pp. 489–490.
38. Markku Linnoila and Matti Virkkunen, "Aggression, Suicidality, and Serotonin," *Journal of Clinical Psychiatry* 53:10 (October 1992 supplement), pp. 46–51.
39. Andreasen, *The Broken Brain*, p. 230.
40. "Genes, Viruses, Hormones and Schizophrenia Etiology," *Clinical Psychiatry News*, August 1992, p. 22.
41. Andreasen, *The Broken Brain*, pp. 185–188.
42. Morton Low, "Evaluation of Psychiatric Disorders and the Effects of Psychotherapeutic and Psychotomimetic Agents," in *Current Practice of Clinical Electroencephalography*, ed. Donald Klass and David Daly (New York: Raven, 1979), pp. 395–410.
43. John Horgan, "Eugenics Revisited," *Scientific American* 268 (June 1993), pp. 122–131.
44. Kaplan and Sadock, *Synopsis of Psychiatry*, p. 79.
45. Larry J. Siever and Kenneth L. Davis, "A Psychobiological Perspective on the Personality Disorders," *American Journal of Psychiatry* 148:12 (December 1991), p. 1648.
46. Tomb, pp. 41–43, 153–155.
47. Eichelman, p. 489.
48. Lishman, pp. 168–171.
49. Arnold Merriam, Alice A. Medalia, and Bernard Wyszynski, "Schizophrenia as a Neurobehavioral Disorder," *Psychiatric Annals* 23:4 (April 1993), pp. 171–174.
50. Richard Restak, "See No Evil," *The Sciences* (July–August 1992), p. 18.
51. Tardiff, p. 495.
52. Tomb, pp. 123–124.
53. Since the 1970s, a syndrome first labeled "episodic dyscon-

trol" and now known as "intermittent explosive disorder" began to draw particular psychiatric interest in the quest to explain human violence as a limbic disturbance. Patients with this diagnosis are prone to sudden assaultive episodes; between paroxysms their behavior remains nonviolent, and they may experience remorse or amnesia for their destructive acts. Affected patients are more likely than the general population to have undergone traumatic births, exhibited behavioral difficulties as children, caused motor vehicle accidents, and shown constitutional sensitivities to alcohol. On laboratory testing, many demonstrate electrical disturbances and other evidence of limbic brain damage.

Sparser data from different patients implicate damage within nonlimbic regions, such as frontal structures that regulate social inhibitions, in the genesis of aggressive behavior. Evidence includes a generally increased but still rough association of violence with seizures, head injuries, abuse during childhood, malnutrition, learning disabilities, diminished IQ, subtle defects on neuropsychological testing, and assorted electroencephalographic abnormalities.

54. Andreasen, *The Broken Brain*, pp. 120–121.
55. Eichelman, p. 489.
56. Merriam *et al.*, pp. 174–177.
57. Restak, "See No Evil," pp. 18, 19.
58. Tardiff, pp. 494–495.
59. Tomb, pp. 122–123.
60. Martin Drooker and Robert Byck, "Physical Disorders Presenting as Psychiatric Illness: A New View," *Psychiatric Times* (July 1992), pp. 19–23.
61. Tomb, pp. 118–120.
62. Frank Ayd, "Novel Antipsychotics, Antidepressants Surveyed in S. F.," *Psychiatric Times* (August 1993), pp. 7–8.
63. Miriam Tucker, "Clozapine-like Antipsychotics Seen as Wave of the Future," *Clinical Psychiatric News* (January 1993), pp. 1, 13.
64. Freedman, p. 862.

65. Jonathan Pincus and Gary Tucker, *Behavioral Neurology* (Oxford: Oxford University Press, 1985), pp. 131, 137–138.
66. Andreasen, *The Broken Brain*, pp. 222, 230.
67. Winson, p. 238.
68. Andreasen, *The Broken Brain*, pp. 136–137.
69. Linda Barr, "Serotonin in Obsessive–Compulsive Disorder," *Psychiatric Times* (July 1993), pp. 24–25.
70. Jeffrey Cummings, "Neurobiological Basis of Obsessive–Compulsive Disorder," *Psychiatric Times* (January 1993), p. 16.
71. Roberto Dominguez, "Serotonergic Antidepressants and Their Efficacy in Obsessive–Compulsive Disorder," *Journal of Clinical Psychiatry* 53:10 (October 1992 supplement), pp. 56–59.
72. Tomb, pp. 75, 79.
73. Siever and Davis, pp. 1648–1650, 1653.
74. Schizotypal personality disorders and frank schizophrenia in particular share common genetic determinants, attentional deficits, eye movement abnormalities, and, during crises, increased dopamine metabolism.

     Among impulsive personality disorders, certain varieties tend to occur in the same families, suggesting a genetic element common to such subtypes. Impulsively antisocial traits correlate with biological indices of an impaired ability to suppress negatively reinforced behaviors; the indices include a reduced sedation threshold, disinhibited motor function, accelerated habituation of skin conductance, and decreased sympathetic response.

     Patients whose personality disturbances involve mood lability exhibit sleep patterns similar to those seen in depression, exaggerated behavioral reactions to drugs that enhance the action of norepinephrine, and improvement after treatment with several other chemicals that affect neurotransmitter function.

     Personality disorders dominated by anxiety show chronically reduced thresholds for sedation, weak habituation, and sympathetic overactivity (Siever and Davis, pp. 1648–1655).
75. Siever and Davis, pp. 1651–1653.

76. De Lecuona *et al.*, pp. 182, 184.
77. Kaplan and Sadock, pp. 72–74.
78. Ross Baldessarini, *Chemotherapy in Psychiatry* (Cambridge: Harvard University Press, 1985), p. 40.
79. Tomb, pp. 25–26.
80. Paul Genova, "Is American Psychiatry Terminally Ill?" *Psychiatric Times* (June 1993), p. 19.
81. Tomb, pp. 26–27.
82. Horgan, p. 127.
83. Capra, p. 120.
84. Unfortunately, the molecular paradigm, applied successfully to the structure of the gene in the 1940s, 1950s, and 1960s, has today become overgeneralized in its application to other areas, including neuropsychiatric research (Capra, pp. 103–104, 113–114, 119–120).
85. Andreasen, *The Broken Brain*, p. 182–183.
86. Kaplan and Sadock, p. 74.
87. Tomb, pp. 42–43, 45–46.
88. It is a gross oversimplification to seek only single causes for any illness. The "single lesion" myth of disease causality arose originally in the germ theories of the nineteenth century, expanded into molecular biology and genetics, and has now been misapplied to the treatment of many multifactorial disease processes. A more balanced view must also account for the fact that the response of a host organism contributes at least as much to pathological states as does the virulence of a noxious agent (Capra, pp. 111, 150, 153–154).
89. Perceptual distortions only indirectly related to brain processes seem to figure strongly in the genesis of aggression. Schizophrenia, mania, cocaine-induced paranoia, and other delusional states number among the most potent identified antecedents of violence. Beyond frank psychosis, simple mismatch between perception and behavioral abilities—producing, for example, frustration in the mentally retarded—can lead to assaultive outbursts. Animal models support these observations in humans: External interference in rats'

ability to smell alters aggressive behavior in experimental contexts.

Social factors correlate with violent behavior. Animal studies suggest that some brain disease processes produce violence only indirectly by changing territorial behavior. The politics of social dominance and even parental input contribute to violence in societies of rodents and primates. Among human psychiatric patients, such factors as institutional settings, interpersonal space, childhood neglect, inappropriate physical restraint, domestic trigger situations, and the psychotherapist's behavior may all play inflammatory roles.

The most powerful predictors of violence in clinical psychiatric practice turn out to be such quasi-tautological factors as previous assaultive history, violent plans, availability of a weapon, and past record of other impulsive behaviors like suicide, sexual promiscuity, profligate spending, property destruction, and reckless driving.

90. Eichelman, pp. 489–490.
91. Restak, "See No Evil," pp. 18–19.
92. Tardiff, pp. 494–498.
93. Freedman, pp. 858–859.
94. Theodore Lidz, "Images in Psychiatry: Adolf Meyer," *American Journal of Psychiatry* 150:7 (July 1993), p. 1098.
95. Owen Flanagan, *The Science of Mind* (Cambridge: M.I.T. Press, 1991), p. 95.
96. Steven Cooper, "Neuroscience in the Future of Psychiatry," *American Journal of Psychiatry* 145:2 (February 1988), p. 272.
97. W. W. Meissner, "The Psychotherapies: Individual, Family, and Group," in Nicholi, ed., *The New Harvard Guide*, p. 463.
98. Tomb, pp. 154–155.
99. Eric Marcus, *Psychosis and Near Psychosis* (New York: Springer-Verlag, 1992), pp. 217–249.
100. Glen Gabbard, Susan Lazar, and Elizabeth Hersh, "Cost-Offset Studies Show Value of Psychotherapy," *Psychiatric Times* (August 1993), p. 21.
101. Yudofsky and Hales, "The Reemergence," p. 4.

102. "Don't Replace Psychotherapy With a Pill, Experts Remind Public-Sector Psychiatrists," *Psychiatric News* (3 July 1992), p. 13.
103. Elio Frattaroli, "The Mind–Body Problem and the Choice of Intervention," *The Psychiatric Times* (November 1991), pp. 75–76.
104. Gabbard *et al.*, p. 21.
105. Restak, "See No Evil," p. 20.
106. American Psychiatric Association, *Biographical Directory* (Washington: American Psychiatric Association, 1989), p. 1573.
107. Thomas Szasz, *The Myth of Mental Illness* (New York: Harper & Row, 1974), p. 262.
108. Frattaroli, p. 73.
109. Genova, p. 20.
110. An extreme example of neuropsychiatric control of patients by doctors occurred in Russia. This was not simply a result of Communist totalitarianism. Balinksy first imported the neuropsychiatric tradition from Greisinger's Germany to St. Petersburg, home of the Russian Tsar, in the nineteenth century. Korsakov, Bekhterev, Sechenov, and Pavlov then promoted neuropsychiatry in pre-Revolutionary Russia. Its hold hardened into stone when the first Russian institute of psychology opened at the University of Moscow in 1911; the institute purposely imported German staff and materialist ideas to use as its own. Though the chaos of the Soviet Revolution in 1917 brought a brief respite of ferment and eclectism, the grip of materialistic dogma soon afterward grew tighter than ever and finally became a stranglehold around psychiatric practice. From then on, classification of psychiatric illnesses in Russia embraced an almost exclusively somatic bias. Its criteria for psychiatric diagnoses included electroencephalographic findings, odd body shapes, and even heart abnormalities. Punitive neuropsychiatric treatments like sulfazine, atropine, and insulin coma were

employed (Mender, notes for a seminar on Soviet psychiatric diagnosis).

111. Capra, pp. 134, 148–149.
112. The early success of chemicals in preventing and curing infectious diseases inspires modern enthusiasm for drug treatment techniques in general; however, confusion abounds regarding the real cause of this success. The decrease in infectious diseases over the last 150 years has stemmed more from general improvement in nutrition and sanitary conditions than from any other factor (Capra, pp. 131–142).
113. Richard Restak, "Brain by Design," *The Sciences* (September–October, 1993), pp. 32–33.
114. Capra, pp. 155, 249.
115. Restak, "Brain by Design," pp. 32–33.
116. Herbert Marcuse, *One-Dimensional Man* (Boston: Beacon Press, 1964), p. 158.
117. Hearnshaw, p. 122.

Chapter 3

1. Donald Palmer, *Does the Center Hold?* (Mountain View: Mayfield, 1991), pp. 18–23.
2. Frattaroli, pp. 73–76.
3. Donald Palmer, *Looking at Philosophy* (Mountain View: Mayfield, 1988), pp. 4–32, 69.
4. Diane Collinson, *Fifty Major Philosophers* (London: Croom Helm, 1987), pp. 17–18.
5. Anthony Flew, *A Dictionary of Philosophy* (New York: St. Martin's Press, 1979), pp. 88, 203.
6. Palmer, *Looking at Philosophy*, pp. 36–37.
7. Stephen Priest, *Theories of the Mind* (Boston: Houghton Mifflin, 1991), p. 99.
8. Hearnshaw, p. 115.
9. Capra, pp. 105–107.

10. Thorne, ed., p. 975.
11. Thomas Hobbes, "Of Sense," in *The Philosophy of Mind*, eds. Brian Beakley and Peter Ludlow (Cambridge: MIT Press, 1992), p. 11.
12. Aviel Goodman, "Organic Unity Theory: The Mind–Body Problem Revisited," *American Journal of Psychiatry* 148:5 (May 1991), p. 554.
13. Palmer, *Looking at Philosophy*, p. 159.
14. Priest, p. 100.
15. Collinson, pp. 51–56.
16. Flew, pp. 150–152.
17. Priest, pp. 100–101.
18. Hearnshaw, pp. 115–116.
19. Thorne, ed., p. 593.
20. Palmer, *Does the Center Hold?* pp. 153–159.
21. Priest, p. 98.
22. Palmer, *Does the Center Hold?* p. 158.
23. U. T. Place, "Is Consciousness a Brain Process?," in Beakley and Ludlow, eds., *The Philosophy of Mind*, pp. 33–39.
24. Priest, pp. 102–115.
25. Epiphenomenalism is said by some to approach a "weak" form of dualism.
26. John Eccles, "A Critical Appraisal of Mind–Brain Theories," in *Cerebral Correlates of Conscious Experience*, eds., Buser and Rougeul-Buser (Oxford: Elsevier, 1978), p. 349.
27. Goodman, p. 554.
28. G. E. Hutchinson, "Man Talking or Thinking," *American Scientist* 64 (January–February 1976), p. 25.
29. Priest, pp. 3–4.
30. Palmer, *Does the Center Hold?* pp. 160–161.
31. Eccles, p. 348.
32. Flanagan, p. 222.
33. Palmer, *Does the Center Hold?* pp. 158–159.
34. Eccles, p. 350.
35. Palmer, *Does the Center Hold?* pp. 352–353.
36. Priest, p. 98.

37. Palmer, *Looking at Philosophy*, pp. 4–32, 69.
38. Flew, pp. 41–44.
39. Bertrand Russell, *A History of Western Philosophy* (New York: Simon and Schuster, 1945), pp. 647–659.
40. Geoffrey Warnock, "Berkeley, George," in Gregory, ed., *The Oxford Companion*, pp. 82–83.
41. Palmer, *Looking at Philosophy*, pp. 36, 192–194.
42. Priest, p. 79.
43. Ibid., pp. 80–97.
44. Collinson, pp. 96–100.
45. Flew, pp. 139–143.
46. Richard Gregory, "Hegel," in Gregory, ed., *The Oxford Companion*, p. 308.
47. Russell, pp. 730–746.
48. Roger Scruton, *From Descartes to Wittgenstein* (New York: Harper & Row, 1982), pp. 165–180.
49. Peter Singer, *Hegel* (Oxford: Oxford University Press, 1983), pp. 1–8.
50. Collinson, pp. 81–86.
51. Gregory, "Hume, David," in Gregory, ed., *The Oxford Companion*, pp. 319–320.
52. Flew, pp, 153–156.
53. Russell, pp. 659–674.
54. Scruton, *From Descartes to Wittgenstein*, pp. 120–133.
55. Collinson, pp. 89–94.
56. John Cottingham, "Kant, Immanuel," in Gregory, ed., *The Oxford Companion*, p. 406.
57. Flew, pp. 189–194.
58. Russell, pp. 701–718.
59. Scruton, *From Descartes to Wittgenstein*, pp. 137–164.
60. Roger Scruton, *Kant* (Oxford: Oxford University Press, 1982), pp. 1–10.
61. Flanagan, pp. 40, 64.
62. Palmer, *Looking at Philosophy*, pp. 192–194.
63. Priest, p. 79.
64. Palmer, *Does the Center Hold?* pp. 181–201.

65. E. T. Bell, *Men of Mathematics* (New York: Simon and Schuster, 1965), pp. 35–52.
66. Collinson, pp. 57–60.
67. John G. Cottingham, "Descartes, René," in Gregory, ed., *The Oxford Companion*, pp. 189–190.
68. Flew, pp. 89–92.
69. Russell, pp. 557–560.
70. Scruton, *From Descartes to Wittgenstein*, pp. 29–49.
71. René Descartes, "Passions of the Soul Brain," in Beakley and Ludlow, eds., *The Philosophy of Mind*, p. 110.
72. Eccles, pp. 351–353.
73. Jerry Fodor, "The Mind–Body Problem," *Scientific American* 244 (January 1981), p. 114.
74. Goodman, pp. 554–555.
75. Hutchinson, p. 25.
76. Scruton, *From Descartes to Wittgenstein*, pp. 123, 125–126.
77. Leibnitz also had mathematical interests and created a computing machine, though his innovations in symbolic logic were overlooked for more than a century and a half. His substantial contributions in developing the calculus were also given short shrift for many years.
78. E. T. Bell, pp. 117–130.
79. Collinson, pp. 57–60.
80. Flanagan, pp. 40, 64.
81. Flew, pp. 198–202.
82. Fodor, p. 114.
83. Goodman, pp. 553, 555.
84. G. W. F. Leibnitz, "Illustrated by the Analogy of the Two Clocks," in Flew, ed., *Body, Mind, and Death*, pp. 152–153.
85. G. MacDonald Ross, *Leibnitz* (Oxford: Oxford University Press, 1984), pp. 3–27.
86. Russell, pp. 581–582.
87. Scruton, *From Descartes to Wittgenstein*, pp. 67–77.
88. Ralph Walker, "Leibnitz, Gottfried Wilhelm, Freiherr Von," in Gregory, ed., *The Oxford Companion*, pp. 57–60.

89. Priest, pp. 85–111.
90. Goodman, pp. 556–558, 561.
91. Flanagan, pp. 14–16, 31, 42–43, 58–62, 217–220.
92. Arthur Koestler, *The Ghost in the Machine* (London: Penguin, 1967), pp. 34, 61–62, 104, 212.
93. Ibid., pp. 50, 64–67, 190, 205, 211, 216–217.
94. Palmer, *Does the Center Hold?* pp. 134, 136–137.
95. Palmer, *Looking at Philosophy*, p. 159.
96. The "wilderness" of endlessly emergent dualisms has its roots in the writings of John Stuart Mill, who alluded to emergence in this philosophy, and of Henri Bergson, who extended emergent concepts specifically to biological evolution. A modern psychiatrist has speculated that current attempts to frame human selfhood within an emergent scheme fuel psychiatry's conceptual "oscillations" (Freedman, pp. 860, 866; Goodman, p. 554; Hearnshaw, p. 121).
97. Eccles, pp. 348–350.
98. Fodor, pp. 116–117.
99. Goodman, pp. 554–561.
100. Palmer, *Looking at Philosophy*, pp. 163–169.
101. Priest, pp. 150–182.
102. Collinson, pp. 69–73.
103. Flew, pp. 334–337.
104. Joanna North, "Spinoza, Benedict (Baruch) de," in Gregory, ed., *The Oxford Companion*, pp. 737–739.
105. Russell, pp. 569–570.
106. Scruton, *From Descartes to Wittgenstein*, pp. 50–66.
107. Baruch Spinoza, "Ethics," in Flew, ed., *Body, Mind, and Death*, p. 146.
108. Erwin Schrödinger, *My View of the World* (Woodbridge: Ox Bow Press, 1983), pp. 43, 214.
109. Eccles, pp. 348–350.
110. Goodman, pp. 554–561.
111. Palmer, *Looking at Philosophy*, pp. 4–32, 69, 163–169.
112. Priest, pp. 150–182.

113. Richard Tarnas, *The Passion of the Western Mind* (New York: Crown, 1981), p. 20.
114. Priest, pp. 22, 155.
115. Flanagan, p. 341.
116. Koestler, p. 201.
117. David Oldroyd, *The Arch of Knowledge* (New York: Methuen 1986), p. 24.
118. Palmer, *Looking at Philosophy*, p. 80.
119. Priest, pp. 81–82.
120. E. T. Bell, pp. 362–377.
121. Edna Kramer, *The Nature and Growth of Modern Mathematics* (Princeton: Princeton University Press, 1981), pp. 368–400.
122. Ibid., pp. 401–433.
123. Ibid., pp. 368–401.
124. Tony Rothman, "The Short Life of Evariste Galois," *Scientific American* 246 (April 1982), pp. 136–149.
125. W. W. Sawyer, *A Concrete Approach to Abstract Algebra* (New York: Dover, 1959), pp. 77–78.
126. Lawrence Sklar, *Space, Time, and Spacetime* (Berkeley: University of California Press, 1976), p. 50.
127. Steven Weinberg, *Dreams of a Final Theory* (New York: Pantheon Books, 1992), p. 3.
128. Herbert Bernstein and Anthony Phillips, "Fiber Bundles and Quantum Theory," *Scientific American* 245 (July 1981), p. 125.
129. P. Davies, *Space and Time in the Modern Universe* (Cambridge: Cambridge University Press, 1977), pp. 9–10.
130. Weinberg, *Dreams of a Final Theory*, p. 3.
131. Richard Feynman, *The Character of Physical Law* (Cambridge: M.I.T. Press, 1965), pp. 84–85.
132. Ibid., pp. 92–94.
133. John Briggs and F. David Peat, *Looking Glass Universe* (New York: Simon and Schuster, 1984), pp. 60–62.
134. Feynman, p. 84.
135. Goodman, p. 561.
136. Hearnshaw, p. 127.
137. Hutchinson, p. 25.

Chapter 4

1. Genova, p. 20.
2. E. T. Bell, pp. 20–24.
3. Collinson, pp. 8–10.
4. Flew, pp. 494–495.
5. "Pythagoras" (no author given), in Gregory, ed., *The Oxford Companion*, p. 665.
6. Kramer, pp. 18–40.
7. Palmer, *Looking at Philosophy*, pp. 16–18.
8. Russell, pp. 29–37.
9. This definition, despite use of the word "one" in the phrase "one-to-one," is not circular. The hyphenated expression, its appearance notwithstanding, does not presuppose the actual concept of a number [Morris Kline, *Mathematics, the Loss of Certainty* (New York: Oxford University Press, 1980), p. 223; Scruton, *From Descartes to Wittgenstein*, pp. 246–247].
10. Collinson, pp. 125–127.
11. Flew, p. 126.
12. Scruton, *From Descartes to Wittgenstein*, p. 241.
13. Flew, pp. 373–374.
14. "Whitehead, Alfred North" (no author given), in Gregory, ed., *The Oxford Companion*, pp. 809–810.
15. Collinson, pp. 134–138.
16. Flew, pp. 308–309.
17. Gregory, "Russell, Bertrand Arthur William," in Gregory, ed., *The Oxford Companion*, pp. 687–688.
18. Palmer, *Looking at Philosophy*, pp. 6–18.
19. Hearnshaw, p. 127.
20. Hutchinson, p. 25.
21. Collinson, p. 61.
22. Kline, p. 234.
23. Kramer, pp. 627–632.
24. Felix Browder, "Does Pure Mathematics Have a Relation to the Sciences?" *American Scientist* 64 (September–October 1976), pp. 546–548.

25. Kline, pp. 192, 198, 227, 248.
26. Capra, pp. 375–376.
27. Collinson, pp. 47–51.
28. Flew, p. 495.
29. Oldroyd, pp. 176–182.
30. "Mach, Ernst" (no author given), in Gregory, ed., *The Oxford Companion*, p. 445.
31. Oldroyd, pp. 231, 234–235.
32. Collinson, pp. 142–144.
33. Oldroyd, p. 232.
34. Hearnshaw, p. 230.
35. Scruton, *From Descartes to Wittgenstein*, p. 278.
36. John Losee, *A Historical Introduction to the Philosophy of Science* (New York: Oxford University Press, 1980), p. 173.
37. Oldroyd, pp. 275–281.
38. Ibid., p. 239.
39. William Kessen and Emily Cahan, "A Century of Psychology: From Subject to Object to Agent," *American Scientist* 24 (November–December 1986), p. 647.
40. Hearnshaw, pp. 226–229, 231.
41. Flanagan, pp. 222–223.
42. Palmer, *Does the Center Hold?* p. 142.
43. Palmer, *Looking at Philosophy*, p. 155.
44. Hearnshaw, pp. 226–227.
45. "Weber, Ernst Heinrich" (no author given), in Gregory, ed., *The Oxford Companion*, pp. 808–809.
46. Fechner's statistical innovations resulted in the methods of average error and of right and wrong cases. His experimental efforts produced a law relating the intensity of a sensation to the logarithm of a stimulus magnitude. The principle led to the acoustic decibel scale and later found parallels in observed relations between light stimulus intensities and evoked neural impulse frequencies. The logarithmic aspect of Fechner's law ultimately gave way to S. S. Stevens's power equation in the 1950s, but Stevens owed his methodology to Fechner's influence (Hearnshaw, pp. 126–129).

47. Capra, pp. 169.
48. O. L. Zangwill, "Fechner, Gustav Theodor," in Gregory, ed., *The Oxford Companion*, pp. 258–259.
49. Hearnshaw, pp. 135, 137, 139–140.
50. Gregory, "Helmholtz, Hermann Ludwig Ferdinand von," Gregory, ed., in *The Oxford Companion*, pp. 308–310.
51. Hearnshaw, pp. 134–137.
52. O. L. Zangwill, "Wundt, Wilhelm Max," in Gregory, ed., *The Oxford Companion*, pp. 816–817.
53. Kessen and Cahan, pp. 641–642.
54. Kerry Buckley, "Watson, John Broadus," in *The Social Science Encyclopedia*, eds. Adam Kuper and Jessica Kuper (New York: Routledge, 1985), pp. 891–892.
55. Robert Epstein, "Watson, John Broadus," in Gregory, ed., *The Oxford Companion*, p. 808.
56. Johnson-Laird, p. 16.
57. Kessen and Cahan, pp. 645–646.
58. Epstein, p. 808.
59. Capra, pp. 175–176.
60. Kessen and Cahan, p. 647.
61. Hearnshaw, pp. 226–227, 230–233.
62. Justin Weiss and Larry Seidman, "The Clinical Use of Psychological and Neuropsychological Tests," in Nicholi, ed., *The New Harvard Guide*, pp. 47, 48, 58.
63. Frattaroli, p. 73.

Chapter 5

1. The mechanistic view of life has found a plentitude of support over the centuries. During the Italian Renaissance, Giovanni Borelli gave a mechanistic spin to selected features of muscle action. The seventeenth-century physiologist William Harvey explained the circulation of blood in the body in terms of hydraulic and anatomical mechanisms. In the eighteenth century, Le Mettrie asserted that the entire human

body operates on mechanical principles. Jacques Loeb's mechanistic biology, put forward in his book *The Mechanistic Conception of Life*, encouraged the idea of behavior as a "tropism", which "forces" movements of organisms through the agency of environmental imperatives. During the early twentieth century, the theory that life functions on a mechanical basis found an advocate in Joseph Needham (Capra, pp. 105–108, 115, 167, 172).

2. Flanagan, pp. 180, 220.
3. Fodor, p. 119.
4. Jeremy Bernstein, *The Analytical Engine* (New York: William Morrow, 1981), p. 71.
5. John Von Neumann, *The Computer and the Brain* (New Haven: Yale University Press, 1958), p. 74.
6. J. Bernstein, p. 112.
7. Robert Heinlein, *The Moon Is a Harsh Mistress* (New York: Ace, 1966), pp. 7–302.
8. Flanagan, pp. 180, 220.
9. Fodor, p. 119.
10. Scott Ladd, *The Computer and the Brain* (New York: Bantam, 1986), pp. 46–47.
11. Robert Hooke first coined the term *cell* in the seventeenth century in response to observations made through the microscope, which had just been invented. Later, the concept of cells as the basic building blocks of life became commonplace among mechanistic biologists. The cell itself was seen to function like a miniature factory (Capra, 109).
12. Digital concepts of mind began with David Hume, who visualized the association of elementary perceptions as a progressive attraction of ideas, an analogy to Newton's force of gravity. Such ideas later became the basis of his so-called "elementist" school of psychology, which in the 1870s asserted that "atomic" perceptual elements and their associations form the basis of mind (Capra, pp. 168–169, 172).
13. Ladd, p. 47.
14. Capra, pp. 168, 169, 173–174.

15. Hearnshaw, pp. 116–119.
16. "Golgi, Camillo" (no author given), in Gregory, ed., *The Oxford Companion*, p. 296.
17. David Hubel, "The Brain," in Gerard Piel *et al.*, eds., *The Brain*, p. 5.
18. "Ramón y Cajal, Santiago" (no author given), in Gregory, ed., *The Oxford Companion*, p. 671.
19. Hearnshaw, pp. 116–119.
20. Georges Thines, "Sherrington, Sir Charles Scott," in Gregory, ed., *The Oxford Companion*, pp. 709–713.
21. Changeux, p. 52.
22. Ibid., p. 31.
23. Ibid., pp. 116–118.
24. Ibid.
25. Mary Brazier, *Electrical Activity of the Nervous System* (Baltimore: Williams and Wilkins, 1977), p. 175.
26. Changeux, pp. 32, 68.
27. Berger was born in 1873. He earned his doctorate in Jena and became a member of the psychiatric staff there. After doing research on spinal cord and brain regulation of blood flow and temperature, Berger entered the army for service during the First World War. He returned to become a professor in Jena and in 1924 began his major investigation, recording the first human electroencephalogram. His findings at the outset found little acceptance, but in 1934, Adrian and Matthews confirmed them in their own studies. Berger went on to try linking brain electricity with mental activity. This work led to his discovery of the so-called "alpha" wave associated with quiescence in the waking state. Berger retired in 1938 but became depressed and committed suicide in 1941.
28. W. Cheyne McCallum, "Berger, Hans," in Gregory, ed., *The Oxford Companion*, p. 81.
29. Adrian was born in 1889 in London. He attended Westminster School and Cambridge, where he earned his degree in medicine and became a professor. He did his postgraduate medical training at St. Bartholomew's Hospital in London

and the National Hospital for Nervous Diseases, Queen Square, in London. He served as a physician in the military during World War I and then again took up research that he had started previously at the Cambridge Physiological Laboratory. There he succeeded in proving the "all-or-nothing" nature of the nerve action potential. Adrian became a world leader in electrophysiological research on nervous tissue, making original discoveries, employing new technologies, and confirming the findings of others like Berger. He wrote a classic monograph entitled *The Basis of Sensation*. He earned the Nobel Prize in 1932 jointly with Sherrington. Lord Adrian became a Baron in 1955 and Chancellor of Cambridge in 1967. He died in 1977.

30. O. L. Zangwill and Y. Zotterman, "Adrian, Edgar Douglas," in Gregory, ed., *The Oxford Companion*, pp. 7–8.
31. Brazier, p. 14.
32. Ladd, 45, 57.
33. Hearnshaw, pp. 116–119, 252–253.
34. Hubel, p. 6
35. Gerard Piel *et al.*, eds., p. 141.
36. Hubel, p. 10.
37. Michael D. Devous, "Imaging Brain Function by Single-Photon Emission Computer Tomography," in Andreasen, ed., *Brain Imaging*, pp. 184–185.
38. Hubel, p. 6.
39. F. H. C. Crick, "Thinking About the Brain," in Gerard Piel *et al.*, eds., *The Brain*, p. 133.
40. Ibid., p. 137.
41. Andreasen, *The Broken Brain*, p. 90.
42. Ibid., p. 219.
43. Frattaroli, p. 76.
44. Andreasen, *The Broken Brain*, p. 219.
45. Ibid., p. 221.
46. The idea of digital genes, both in their early abstract form and later as concrete biochemical entities embodied in the molecules of DNA, changed conceptions of the basic units of

life. These units were thought to be cells in the nineteenth century but genes in the twentieth. Thus, Gregor Mendel's initial discovery that genes and observable traits exhibit a one-to-one correspondence led to the ultimate notion of genes as computable "bits" of heredity (Capra, pp. 113–114, 116).

47. Flanagan, p. 269, 292–293, 300.
48. Hearnshaw, p. 258.
49. Johnson-Laird, p. 50.
50. Koestler, pp. 115, 159–160.
51. The pioneering ethological field studies of Konrad Lorenz and Niko Tinbergen showed that many innate behaviors in animals are inherited and exhibit features associated with constitutionally fixed mechanisms. Further support for the ethological viewpoint came from some human behaviors that appear not to vary in different cultural contexts. Ethology thus acquired the authority to inspire Bowlby's psychiatric work on the origin of human mental illness in maternal deprivation during innately determined critical periods of infant development (Hearnshaw, pp. 142, 258–262).
52. Calvin Hall introduced quantitative elements into the discipline of psychogenetics. In 1951, he advocated controlled animal breeding experiments to tease out behavioral differences among genetic strains. Fuller and Thompson expanded this idea in 1960 to include statistical analysis of inherited behavioral patterns in human populations as well. Spinoff projects evolved, including Freeman's comparisons of behaviors in separated twins and foster children. Such data prompted psychiatrists to conclude that "studies of twins . . . reared apart . . . demonstrate a major genetic influence on personality development. . . ." Burt's multifactorial analysis applied to inheritance of intellect and chromosome studies of anomalies in intelligence also appeared in the research literature. Other researchers studied the genetic shaping of aggressive behavior through animal breeding experiments as well as human family behavior patterns

(Eichelman, p. 489; Hearnshaw, pp. 256–257; Siever and Davis, p. 1648).

53. Hearnshaw, pp. 19, 141, 143.
54. D. R. D., "Morgan, Conwy Lloyd," in Gregory, ed., *The Oxford Companion*, p. 496.
55. Hearnshaw, pp. 141, 143.
56. O. L. Zangwill, "Jackson, John Hughlings," in Gregory, ed., *The Oxford Companion*, p. 395.
57. Flanagan, p. 325.
58. Koestler, pp. 98, 275, 286–287, 289.
59. Charles Hampden-Turner, *Maps of the Mind* (New York: Collier Books, 1982), p. 80.
60. Freedman, p. 865.
61. Hampden-Turner, pp. 80–83.
62. Hearnshaw, p. 119.
63. Francois Jacob, *The Possible and the Actual* (New York: Pantheon, 1982), pp. 36–37.
64. Koestler, pp. 273, 281–284, 299, 319–322, 332.
65. Thorne, ed., p. 122.
66. Hearnshaw, p. 118.
67. "Cannon, Walter Bradford" (no author given), in Gregory, ed., *The Oxford Companion*, p. 125.
68. Hearnshaw, p. 250
69. Andreasen, *The Broken Brain*, pp. 121–122.
70. Hearnshaw, pp. 248, 253, 255.
71. Koestler, p. 98.
72. Winson, pp. 42–43.
73. Crick, pp. 134, 136.
74. Flanagan, pp. 226, 231.
75. Crick, p. 134.
76. Ibid.
77. Changeux, p. 19.
78. Ladd, pp. 44–45.
79. Following the lead of rabies researchers, physiologists tried to firm up links between violent behavior and abnormal electrical activity in limbic brain structures as well as neighboring

areas like the hypothalamus and mesial temporal lobe. It became known that experimental damage to septal nuclei in the rat's limbic system increases defensive behavior, that injury to a related part of the hypothalamus augments offensive activity, and that other maneuvers affect predatory aggression.

80. Eichelman, pp. 488, 494.
81. Restak, "See No Evil," p. 18.
82. Winson, p. 242.
83. Andreasen, *The Broken Brain*, pp. 108–109.
84. Gerard Piel *et al.*, eds., p. 142.
85. Sandra Witelson, "Cognitive Neuroanatomy," *Neurology* 42 (April 1992), p. 709.
86. Hearnshaw, p. 255.
87. Witelson, pp. 709, 711.
88. Justin Weiss and Larry Seidman, "The Clinical Use of Tests," in Nicholi, ed., *The New Harvard Guide*, p. 47.
89. Sandra Weintraub and M. Marsel Mesulam, "Mental State Assessment of Young and Elderly Adults in Behavioral Neurology," in *Principles of Behavioral Neurology*, ed. M. Marsel Mesulam (Philadelphia: F. A. Davis, 1985), p. 76–123.
90. Andreasen, *The Broken Brain*, pp. 108, 172–173.
91. Mender, CT, MRI, PET scanning lecture notes.
92. Crick, p. 132–133.
93. Changeux, pp. 16, 17, 21.
94. Freedman, pp. 863–864.

Chapter 6

1. Winson, p. 23.
2. Flanagan, pp. 226, 231.
3. Paul Wallich, "Silicon Babies," *Scientific American* 265 (December 1991), pp. 124–134.
4. Jacob Bronowski, *The Origins of Knowledge and Imagination* (New Haven: Yale University Press, 1978), p. 14.

5. Crick, pp. 131–132.
6. Jonathan Cohen and David Servan-Schreiber, "Introduction to Neural Network Models in Psychiatry," *Psychiatric Annals* 22:3 (March 1922), p. 115.
7. Ralph Hoffman, "Attractor Neural Networks and Psychotic Disorders," *Psychiatric Annals* 22:3 (March 1992), p. 120.
8. Hubel, p. 4.
9. Ladd, pp. x, 39–41, 57–63, 66, 72, 74–76.
10. Bernard Williams, "Leviathan's Program," *New York Review of Books* (11 June 1987), p. 33.
11. R. Hoffman, pp. 119–120.
12. Cohen and Servan-Schreiber, pp. 114–115.
13. These statistical properties are connected with action potential frequency characteristics and with the theoretical sample spaces of probabilistic machines.
14. Hubel, p. 6.
15. Mark Kac, "Probability," *Scientific American* 211 (September 1964), pp. 96–100.
16. Priest, pp. 139–141.
17. Von Neumann, pp. 76–78.
18. Jacob Bronowski, *The Identity of Man* (Garden City: The Natural History Press, 1966), p. 34.
19. Ladd, pp. 95–120.
20. Cohen and Servan-Schreiber, p. 115.
21. Crick, pp. 131–132.
22. Cortical sensors in mammals, for instance, send signals not only to the frontal lobe, but also to the hippocampus, the neurons of which form a crazy quilt of connections with structures such as the motor cortex, basal ganglia, and amygdala; several, including the amygdala, send reciprocal signals back to the hippocampus.
23. Crick, p. 135.
24. Cohen and Servan-Schreiber, p. 115.
25. Martha Farah and James McClelland, "Neural Network Models and Cognitive Neuropsychology," *Psychiatric Annals* 22:3 (March 1922), pp. 148–149, 153.

26. Hubel, p. 9.
27. Ladd, p. 111.
28. Michael Arbib, "McCulloch, Walter Sturgis," in Gregory, ed., *The Oxford Companion*, p. 443.
29. Crick, p. 136.
30. Ladd, pp. 28–29.
31. Michael Arbib and Richard Gregory, "McCulloch's Contributions to Brain Theory," in Gregory, ed., *The Oxford Companion*, pp. 443–444.
32. Johnson-Laird, p. 355.
33. Flourens' work in the early nineteenth century debunked Franz Gall's primitive localization ideas. Gall, who was born in 1758 and worked as a physician in Vienna, claimed that feeling the lumps on people's heads tells something about their psychological makeup. He blamed particular mental functions residing in specific brain sites for skull overgrowth, cited experimental proof, and thus presaged later localization theories in neuropsychiatry. Despite thin supportive data, his "phrenology" won over a student, Johann Kaspar Spurzheim, and a Scottish philosopher, George Combe, who became proselytizers on Gall's behalf. A total of 35 traits, including combativeness, self-esteem, hope, wonder, and wit, were assigned addresses on the skull by Gall and his disciples. By 1832, 29 phrenological societies existed in Britain alone. Gall's views fell into disfavor when Flourens tested Gall's ideas in animal models (Gregory, "Phrenology," Gregory, ed., in *The Oxford Companion*, pp. 618–620).
34. Changeux, pp. 13–17.
35. O. L. Zangwill, "Gall, Sir Francis," in Gregory, ed., *The Oxford Companion*, p. 282.
36. Hearnshaw, pp. 116–119.
37. O. L. Zangwill, "Lashley, Karl Spencer," in Gregory, ed., *The Oxford Companion*, pp. 427–428.
38. Ibid., p. 428.
39. Ibid., pp. 427–428.
40. Crick, p. 134.

41. Flanagan, pp. 232–235, 316.
42. Johnson-Laird, p. 178.
43. Emmett N. Leith and Juris Upatnieks, "Photography by Laser," *Scientific American* 212 (June 1965), pp. 24–35.
44. Karl Pribram, "The Neurophysiology of Remembering," *Scientific American* 220 (January 1969), pp. 73–86.
45. Flanagan, pp. 239–240.
46. Vernon Mountcastle, ed., *Medical Physiology*, Vol. 1 (St. Louis: Mosby, 1980), p. iii.
47. Brazier, pp. 118–120.
48. Changeux, pp. 58, 122.
49. Ladd, p. 47.
50. Hubel, born in Windsor, Ontario, was educated as a physician at McGill University and as a neurological specialist at the Montreal Neurological Institute and Johns Hopkins Hospital. In 1955, he began a research career in neurophysiology, first at the Walter Reed Army Institute of Research and then at Johns Hopkins and Harvard (Gerard Piel *et al.*, eds., p. 141).
51. Wiesel, born in Sweden, earned his medical degree at the Karolinska Institute in Stockhom. In the mid-1950s, he began collaborating with Hubel after becoming a faculty member at Johns Hopkins. Wiesel, like Hubel, later moved to Harvard and also became chairman of its neurobiology department (Gerard Piel *et al.*, eds., pp. 141–142).
52. H. B., "Hubel and Wiesel: Joint Work," in Gregory, ed., *The Oxford Companion*, pp. 313–315.
53. Winson, pp. 27–31, 185–186, 242.
54. Ladd, pp. 67, 91.
55. Cohen and Servan-Schreiber, pp. 114, 117.
56. Ibid., pp. 115–117.
57. Ibid., p. 117.
58. R. Hoffman, pp. 120–121.
59. David Li and David Spiegel, "A Neural Network Model of Dissociative Disorders," *Psychiatric Annals* 22:3 (March 1922), pp. 145–146.

60. Jeffrey Sutton, Adam Mamelak, and J. Allan Hobson, "Modeling States of Waking and Sleeping," *Psychiatric Annals* 22:3 (March 1922), p. 141.
61. Cohen and Servan-Schreiber, pp. 116–117.
62. Sutton *et al.*, pp. 138, 142.
63. Cohen and Servan-Schreiber, p. 115.
64. David Servan-Schreiber and Jonathan Cohen, "A Neural Network Model of Catecholamine Modulation of Behavior," *Psychiatric Annals* 22:3 (March 1922), pp. 125–127, 129.
65. Sutton *et al.*, p. 137.
66. The modulating substance dopamine begins life in the midbrain, and its cells of origin project it to the frontal brain surface. Particular focus of dopamine's gain-sharpening actions on specific feedback loops in the forebrain apparently enables it to match behavior with changing stimulus contexts.

Norepinephrine and serotonin originate in cells within the brain's base or "stem." Both substances exert active modulating influences on the entire surface of the brain during wakefulness, sharpening its signal-to-noise ratio. Norepinephrine activity increases especially in response to alerting or noxious stimulation. This serves to further enhance signal-to-noise discriminatory abilities of the conscious brain during unexpected, threatening situations requiring fight or flight responses.

Acetylcholine, originating from cell groups located in both the brainstem and forebrain, has modulating effects that do not sharpen gain. Instead, acetylcholine increases the sensitivity but not the selectivity of neuronal unit activation. This influence increases the output of forebrain cells in response to excitatory stimuli without exaggerating inhibition. As a result, modulating influences produce diffuse, indiscriminate output irritability consistent with the cognitive incoherence of sleep. During wakefulness, acetylcholine activity remains sparse and increases only in response to novel input stimuli. With descent into non-dreaming sleep, a steady output increase of acetylcholine issues from the brain-stem. During dreams, periodic, inconstant bursts of cholinergic modulation produce characteristic waveforms in electrical recordings.

Hence, a mechanistic picture of sleep–wake cycles that would please any neuropsychiatrist emerges from the rhythmic, oscillating interactions among the various chemical modulatory systems. This picture also seems to explain why the core of the brainstem, when directly stimulated by artificial means, produces behavioral and neuroelectrical changes identical to those seen during spontaneous arousal. Connectionistic concepts of neuromodulation suggest that alerting involves serotonin and norepinephrine originating in the brainstem, with extreme arousal accompanied especially by release of the latter substance. Acetylcholine also seems to play some role in diffuse aspects of intense arousal but exerts more pervasive and profound effects as the brain descends into sleep, particularly during dreams [Blakeslee, "Scientists Unraveling Chemistry of Dreams," *The New York Times* (7 January 1992), pp. C1, C10; Cohen and Servan-Schreiber, "A Neural Network Model of Disturbances in the Processing of Context in Schizophrenia," *Psychiatric Annals* 22:3 (March 1922), pp. 131–133; Sutton *et al.*, pp. 137–142; Daniel Weinberger, "A Connectionist Approach to the Prefrontal Cortex," *Journal of Neuropsychiatry* 5:3 (Summer 1993), pp. 241–253].

67. Servan-Schreiber and Cohen, pp. 126–129.
68. Ibid., p. 125.
69. Li and Spiegel, pp. 144–146.
70. Ladd, pp. 111–114.
71. Kevin J. Connolly, "Genetics of Behavior," in Gregory, ed., *The Oxford Companion*, p. 284.
72. Winson, pp. 173, 220.
73. Cohen and Servan-Schreiber, pp. 131–135.
74. R. Hoffman, pp. 121–122.
75. Cohen and Servan-Schreiber, pp. 131–135.
76. R. Hoffman, pp. 123–124.

77. Flanagan, pp. 328–330, 333, 346.
78. The ordered chaos of brain processes also reveals itself in the ubiquity of a common though irregular electrical wave signal throughout the overall neural network, even in the absence of a driving stimulus. This self-organizing feature typifies the behavior of chaotic systems.
79. Walter Freeman, "The Physiology of Perception," *Scientific American* 264 (February 1991), pp. 78–79, 82–85.
80. Hartmut Jurgens, Heinz-Otto Peitgen, and Dietmar Saupe, "The Language of Fractals," *Scientific American* 263 (August 1990), pp. 60–67.
81. Stuart Kauffman, "Antichaos and Adaptation," *Scientific American* 265 (August 1991), pp. 78–84.
82. Barry Madore and Wendy Freedman, "Self-organizing Structures," *American Scientist* 75 (May–June 1987), pp. 252–259.
83. Hubel, p. 10.
84. Ladd, p. 9.
85. Freeman, pp. 78–82.
86. Johnson-Laird, p. 193.
87. Ibid., p. 354.
88. Michael Lockwood, *Mind, Brain and the Quantum* (Oxford: Basil Blackwood, 1989), p. 247.
89. Ibid., p. 248.
90. Capra, p. 376.

Chapter 7

1. Ladd, p. 98.
2. J. Bernstein, p. 71.
3. Bronowski, *The Origins of Knowledge and Imagination*, p. 84.
4. Jacob Bronowski, *A Sense of the Future* (Cambridge: M.I.T. Press, 1977), p. 65.
5. Kline, p. 204.
6. Jacob Bronowski, *Magic, Science, and Civilization* (New York: Columbia University Press, 1978), p. 77.

7. Kline, pp. 221–222.
8. Koestler, p. 34.
9. Kline, pp. 190, 199.
10. Flew, p. 296.
11. Though delineating a class through some universal defining property can create paradoxes, overall definitions also have advantages. They can handle infinite sets not tractable through definitions that simply list a finite number of constituent class elements.
12. Kline, pp. 187, 199, 201, 203, 205, 212, 217, 221.
13. Scruton, *From Descartes to Wittgenstein*, pp. 245–246.
14. Flew, pp. 349–350.
15. Mary Elizabeth Tiles, "Gödel, Kurt," in Gregory, ed., *The Oxford Companion*, pp. 294–295.
16. "Turing, Alan Mathison" (no author given), in Gregory, ed., *The Oxford Companion*, pp. 783–784.
17. Douglas Hofstadter, *Gödel, Escher, Bach* (New York: Vintage, 1979), pp. 594–595.
18. These quandaries relate to the vain formalistic project of constructing an axiomatic system tightly enough to avoid inconsistencies yet loosely enough to encompass all of mathematics. The entire enterprise has proven unable to achieve either goal. Its double failure is mirrored in Gödel's restrictions on axiomatic completeness and in the so-called Lowenheim–Skolem theorem, which allows multiple interpretations of undefined terms in mathematics.
19. Max Delbruck, *Mind from Matter?* (Palo Alto: Blackwell, 1986), pp. 177–183.
20. Kline, pp. 176, 181, 191, 227–228, 255, 261, 263, 267–268, 271–273.
21. William Barrett, *The Death of the Soul* (Garden City: Doubleday, 1986), p. 68.
22. J. Bernstein, p. 112.
23. Bronowski, *A Sense of the Future*, pp. 65, 82.
24. Flanagan, p. 215.
25. Kline, p. 263.

26. Palmer, *Does the Center Hold?* pp. 124, 344.
27. Palmer, *Looking at Philosophy*, pp. 178, 309, 331–338, 358.
28. Scruton, *From Descartes to Wittgenstein*, p. 247.
29. Bronowski, *A Sense of the Future*, p. 62.
30. Palmer, *Looking at Philosopher*, pp. 202–204.
31. Erwin Schrödinger, *What Is Life?/Mind and Matter* (Cambridge: Cambridge University Press, 1967), p. 157.
32. Scruton, *From Descartes to Wittgenstein*, pp. 125–126.
33. Dick Teresi, "Perhaps This Universe Is Only a Test," *New York Times Book Review* (5 September 1993), p. 11.
34. Browder, "Does Pure Mathematics Have a Relation to the Sciences?" p. 549.
35. Marcuse, *One-Dimensional Man*, pp. 145–146, 152, 157, 162–163.
36. Vaclav Havel, "The End of the Modern Era," *New York Times* (1 March 1992), p. E15.
37. Marcuse, *One-Dimensional Man*, p. xiv.
38. Frattaroli, pp. 73–74.
39. Briggs and Peat, pp. 24–32.
40. David Bloor, "Kuhn, Thomas Samuel," in Kuper and Kuper, eds., *The Social Science Encyclopedia*, pp. 432–433.
41. Losee, p. 203.
42. Oldroyd, pp. 320–327.
43. Bronowski, *The Origins of Knowledge and Imagination*, pp. 46–47.
44. Bronowski, *A Sense of the Future*, pp. 46, 86–87, 90.
45. Ibid., p. 39.
46. Martin Gardner, "WAP, SAP, PAP & FAP: The Anthropic Cosmological Principle," *New York Review of Books* (May 8, 1986), pp. 22–25.
47. Bronowski, *The Identity of Man*, p. 34.
48. Ibid., pp. 132–133.
49. Hearnshaw, pp. 226–227, 230–233.
50. Kessen and Cahan, p. 647.
51. Bronowski, *The Identity of Man*, p. 78.
52. Hearnshaw, pp. 128, 132, 136–137.

53. Harold Morowitz, *The Wine of Life* (New York: Bantam, 1979), p. 148.
54. Hubel, p. 9.
55. Ladd, p. 54.
56. Winson, p. 188.
57. Ladd, pp. 4–5.
58. Kandel, pp. 1033–1036.
59. Eric Kandel, "Environmental Determinants of Brain Architecture and of Behavior: Early Experience and Learning," in *Principles of Neural Science*, eds. Eric Kandel and James Schwartz (New York: Elsevier, 1981), pp. 625–631.
60. Gregory Chaitin, "Randomness and Mathematic Proof," *Scientific American* 232 (May 1975), pp. 47–52.
61. Capra, pp. 123, 132, 143–144.
62. David Gelman, Debra Rosenberg, Paul Kandell, and Rebecca Crandall, "Is the Mind an Illusion?" *Newsweek* (20 April 1992), pp. 71–72.
63. Gregory, ed., *The Oxford Companion*, p. x.
64. Ibid., p. xi.
65. Daniel Dennett and John C. Haugeland, "Intentionality," in Gregory, ed., *The Oxford Companion*, p. 383.
66. Palmer, *Looking at Philosophy*, p. 361.
67. Dennett and Haugeland, p. 383.
68. Intentionality has roots going back to Aristotle. Medieval Scholastics such as Saint Thomas Aquinas coined the actual term from a Latin word that means "to point at" or "extend toward." More modern ways to address intentionality include "hermeneutic" modes of inquiry, which approach their subject matter as an interpretable "text" concealing levels of meaning that require imaginative commentary. The latter perspective forms the basis for work by such philosophers as Nietzsche, Heidegger, Gadamer, Feyerabend, Derrida, Kuhn, and, to some extent, Freud [Flanagan, p. 28; Quentin Skinner, ed., *The Return of Grand Theory in the Human Sciences* (Cambridge: Cambridge University Press, 1985), pp. 6–7, 10].

69. Flanagan, pp. 62, 179.
70. Hearnshaw, pp. 233–237, 239–243.
71. Flanagan, p. 179.
72. Ibid., p. 29.
73. John Searle, *Minds, Brains and Science* (Cambridge: Harvard University Press, 1984), p. 39.
74. Flanagan, p. 376.
75. Flew, pp. 48–49.
76. Hearnshaw, p. 234.
77. Georges Thines, "Brentano, Franz," in Gregory, ed., *The Oxford Companion*, pp. 117–118.
78. Franz Brentano, *Psychology from an Empirical Standpoint*, as quoted in Hearnshaw, p. 234.
79. Flanagan, pp. 62, 179.
80. Searle, *Minds, Brains and Sciences*, p. 39.
81. Flanagan, p. 30.
82. Ibid., p. 29.
83. John Searle, "Is the Brain's Mind a Computer Program?" *Scientific American* 262 (January 1990), p. 27.
84. Hearnshaw, pp. 240–241
85. George Kerner, *Three Philosophical Moralists* (Oxford: Clarendon, 1990), p. 172.
86. William Barrett, *The Illusion of Technique* (Garden City: Anchor, 1976), p. 131.
87. Bronowski, *A Sense of the Future*, p. 71.
88. Eccles, p. 348.
89. Flanagan, p. 336.
90. Goodman, p. 559.
91. Crick, p. 136.
92. Fodor, pp. 107, 122.
93. Ladd, pp. 28–29, 31.
94. Hearnshaw, p. 272.
95. "Babbage, Charles" (no author given), in Gregory, ed., *The Oxford Companion*, p. 68.
96. Frank George, "Wiener, Norbert," in Gregory, ed., *The Oxford Companion*, pp. 810–811.

97. J. F. Young, *Information Theory* (New York: Wiley, 1971), pp. 1–38.
98. Flanagan, p. 29.
99. Hearnshaw, pp. 240–241.
100. Searle, "Is the Brain's Mind a Computer Program?" p. 26.
101. Hearnshaw, pp. 240–241.
102. Searle, "Is the Brain's Mind a Computer Program?," p. 28.
103. Hearnshaw, pp. 275, 293.
104. Flanagan, pp. 107–109, 237.
105. Johnson-Laird, pp. 184–190.
106. Palmer, *Does the Center Hold?* p. 152.
107. Johnson-Laird, p. 354.
108. Bronowski, *The Identity of Man*, p. 19.
109. Mario Bunge, *Causality and Modern Science* (New York: Dover, 1979), pp. 309–350.
110. Roger Penrose, *The Emperor's New Mind* (Oxford: Oxford University Press, 1989), pp. 243, 248, 249–251, 269–270, 288, 295–298.
111. Lawrence Wile, "Quantum Concepts," *Psychiatric Times* (February 1993), p. 9.
112. John Searle, "Minds and Brains without Programs," in *Mindwaves*, eds., Colin Blakemore and Susan Greenfield (Oxford: Basil Blackwell, 1987), pp. 209–210.
113. Flanagan, p. 258.

Chapter 8

1. Bronowski, *A Sense of the Future*, p. 61.
2. Capra, pp. 375–376.
3. Browder, pp. 546–548.
4. Kline, p. 228.
5. Bronowski, *A Sense of the Future*, p. 61.
6. Martin Davis and Reuben Hersh, "Nonstandard Analysis," *Scientific American* 226 (June 1972), pp. 78–86.
7. Philip Davis and Reuben Hersh, *The Mathematical Experience* (Boston: Houghton Miflin, 1981), pp. 237–254.

8. Kline, pp. 274–275.

9. Lynn Arthur Steen, "New Models of the Real Number Line," *Scientific American* 225 (August 1971), pp. 92–99.

10. Paul Cohen and Reuben Hersh, "Non-Cantorian Set Theory," *Scientific American* 217 (December 1967), pp. 104–116.

11. P. Davis and Hersh, pp. 237–254.

12. Delbruck, p. 166.

13. Kline, pp. 268–270.

14. Steen, pp. 92–99.

15. Andrew Coleman, "Neumann, John von," in Kuper and Kuper, eds., *The Social Science Encyclopedia*, p. 558.

16. Frank George, "Von Neumann, John," in Gregory, ed., *The Oxford Companion*, pp. 804–805.

17. Von Neumann, pp. 81–82.

18. Bronowski, *A Sense of the Future*, pp. 61–62.

19. Albert Einstein and Leopold Infeld, *The Evolution of Physics* (New York: Simon and Schuster, 1966), pp. 125, 143, 146–147.

20. Schellenberg, pp. 63–86.

21. Sawyer, pp. 32–33, 186–187.

22. Janjit Singh, *Great Ideas of Modern Mathematics* (New York: Dover, 1959), pp. 143, 146, 150–152, 157.

23. Donald Davidson, "Mental Events," in Beakley and Ludlow, eds., *The Philosophy of Mind*, pp. 30–149.

24. Davidson concludes from this insight that assertions associated with mind–brain identity theories cannot all be true in their classical forms. He lists three such assertions; to reconcile them all, he deems it necessary to assume that absolute laws of psychophysics cannot be formulated. In this respect, he moves in a direction analogous to that taken by Einstein when he invoked relativistic notions of spatial curvature in order to surmount Kant's mutually contradictory "antinomies" of space [J. J. Callahan, "The Curvature of Space in a Finite Universe," *Scientific American* 235 (August 1976), pp. 90–100; Flew, pp. 83–84].

25. Priest, pp. 115–122.

26. Goodman, pp. 556–559.

27. Daniel Z. Freedman and Peter van Nieuwenhuizen, "Supergravity and the Unification of the Laws of Physics," *Scientific American* 238 (February 1978), pp. 134–135.
28. Bernstein and Phillips, p. 130.
29. Freedman and van Nieuwenhuizen, pp. 134–135.
30. Ibid.
31. Kramer, pp. 632–638.
32. Gerard t'Hooft, "Gauge Theories of the Forces between Elementary Particles," *Scientific American* 242 (June 1980), p. 112.
33. Bernstein and Phillips, pp. 133–137.
34. t'Hooft, pp. 110, 112–116.
35. Sklar, pp. 13–17.
36. Barrett, *The Illusion of Technique*, p. 131.
37. Flanagan, p. 29.
38. Hearnshaw, pp. 240–241.
39. Kerner, p. 172.
40. Quentin Skinner, ed., "Introduction," in *The Return of Grand Theory*, pp. 6–7, 205.
41. Sklar, pp. 40–42.
42. Flanagan, p. 97.
43. Scruton, *From Descartes to Wittgenstein*, pp. 248–249.
44. William Barrett, *Irrational Man* (New York: Doubleday, 1958), pp. 161–163, 210, 230–231, 235.
45. Oldroyd, p. 20.
46. Palmer, *Does the Center Hold?* pp. 155–156, 171–173, 187.
47. Palmer, *Looking at Philosophy*, pp. 251, 349, 365.
48. Immanuel Kant, *Critique of Pure Reason*, as quoted in Palmer, *Does the Center Hold?* p. 187.
49. Ibid.
50. A. D'Abro, *The Rise of the New Physics*, vol. 1 (New York: Dover, 1951), pp. 37–40.
51. Y. I. Manin, *Mathematics and Physics* (Boston: Birkauser, 1981), p. 43.
52. Flanagan, pp. 44, 46.
53. Edmund Whitaker has dramatized this crucial feature of the creative scientific process by showing that most scientific

assertions can best be stated as "laws of the impossible" or "postulates of impotence." Such negative restatements, for example, reduce the laws of mechanics to dicta forbidding perpetual motion. They boil down electromagnetic theory to the idea that the inside of a hollow conductor cannot induce an electric field. They summarize special relativity as the impossibility of detecting uniform speed, general relativity as the absurdity of distinguishing gravity from accelerated motion, and quantum physics as the uncertainty of experimental measurement at the atomic level.

54. Karl Popper, *Unended Quest* (Glasgow: Collins, 1976), p. 79.
55. Bronowski, *A Sense of the Future*, pp. 55, 227–228.
56. W. Bartley, "Popper, Karl Raimund," in Kuper and Kuper, eds., *The Social Science Encyclopedia*, p. 621.
57. Flew, pp. 281–282.
58. Losee, p. 160.
59. Oldroyd, pp. 297–317.
60. R. A. Fisher's statistical concept of the "null hypothesis" combines *modus tollens* reasoning with numerical measurement (Hearnshaw, p. 232).
61. Oldroyd, pp. 26, 45, 301–304.
62. Flanagan, pp. 78, 81.
63. Koestler, p. 156.
64. Popper, p. 79.
65. Bronowski, *The Origins of Knowledge and Imagination*, p. 109.
66. Bronowski, *A Sense of the Future*, pp. 95, 100.
67. Flanagan, p. 125.
68. Manin, pp. 18, 19.
69. Bronowski, *A Sense of the Future*, p. 91.
70. Losee, pp. 168, 187.
71. t'Hooft, pp. 136–138.
72. Oldroyd, pp. 14, 22.
73. Tarnas, p. 10.
74. Flanagan, pp. 143–144.
75. Ibid., pp. 73, 124–125, 131, 183, 187, 192–193, 340.
76. Palmer, *Does the Center Hold?* p. 51.

77. Palmer, *Looking at Philosophy*, pp. 202–204.
78. Roger Penrose, "The Geometry of the Universe," in *Mathematics Today*, ed. Lynn Arthur Steen (New York: Random House, 1978), pp. 85–89.
79. Phillip Rieff, *Freud: The Mind of the Moralist*, quoted in Hans Eysenck, *Decline and Fall of the Freudian Empire* (New York: Penguin 1985), p. 196.

Chapter 9

1. Searle, *Minds, Brains and Science*, pp. 39, 60.
2. Palmer, *Does the Center Hold?* p. 71.
3. Penrose, *The Emperor's New Mind*, pp. 335–339.
4. Stuart Shapiro and Saul Teukolsky, "Black Holes, Naked Singularities and Cosmic Censorship," *American Scientist* 79 (July–August, 1991), pp. 330–343.
5. Physical gauge fields can include not only cusplike singularities but also other anomalies resembling plateaus and jug handles. Analogies to these additional structures, in the setting of an intentional gauge field, might conceivably represent nonpsychotic mental disturbances like neuroses and personality disorders. They may therefore merit further investigation.
6. Capra, pp. 171, 377–381.
7. Michel Foucault, *Mental Illness and Psychology* (Berkeley: University of California Press, 1987), p. 27.
8. A. J. Ayer, *Philosophy in the Twentieth Century* (New York: Vintage 1982), p. 214.
9. Collinson, pp. 128–130.
10. Flew, p. 157.
11. Scruton, *From Descartes to Wittgenstein*, pp. 257–259.
12. Flanagan, p. 178.
13. Hearnshaw, p. 234.
14. Herbert Marcuse, *Negations* (London: Free Association Books, 1988), pp. 58–60.
15. Priest, 198–199, 207.

16. Robert Solomon, *Continental Philosophy Since 1750* (Oxford: Oxford University Press, 1988), pp. 129–138.

17. Hannah Arendt, *The Life of the Mind* (New York: Harcourt Brace Jovanovich, 1978), p. 46.

18. Marcuse, *Negations*, pp. 58–60.

19. Priest, pp. 198–199, 207.

20. F. David Peat, *Superstrings and the Search for the Theory of Everything* (Chicago: Contemporary Books, 1988), p. 225.

21. Penrose, "The Geometry of the Universe," in Steen, ed., *Mathematics Today*, pp. 108–109.

22. If the elemental "point" in an intentional gauge field is ontic in character, then that point's expansion into a torsional "line may correspond to Heidegger's concept of self-transcendent existence or *Dasein* (Barrett, *Irrational Man*, pp. 218–222, 226).

23. Peat, pp. 163–273.

24. Penrose, "The Geometry of the Universe," pp. 122–124.

25. Roger Penrose, "Minds, Machines and Mathematics," in Blakemore and Greenfield, eds., *Mindwaves*, p. 274.

26. Peat, pp. 168–169.

27. Palmer, *Looking at Philosophy*, p. 361.

28. Priest, pp. 82, 208–209.

29. Barrett, *The Death of the Soul*, pp. 44–46.

30. Palmer, *Looking at Philosophy*, pp. 204–205.

31. Scruton, *From Descartes to Wittgenstein*, p. 128.

32. Barrett, *The Death of the Soul*, pp. 64, 114–115.

33. Scruton, *From Descartes to Wittgenstein*, p. 147.

34. Palmer, *Looking at Philosophy*, pp. 222–234.

35. Priest, pp. 80–97.

36. Scruton, *From Descartes to Wittgenstein*, pp. 165–180.

37. Barrett, *The Death of the Soul*, p. 116.

38. The rising accord given to neutral monism in modern thought has heightened this blurring. Some modern versions of neutral monism have even tried to replace numbers with the self as their invariant, leading to new variations on the infinite regressions of global epistemic symmetry (Priest, pp. 170–182).

39. Goodman, pp. 554–558.
40. Koestler, p. 58.
41. Capra, p. 373.
42. A threefold approach to representations of reality is not new. Karl Popper, for example, has advocated his own "three-world" metaphysical construct, consisting not of a simple matter–mind dualism but instead of physics, consciousness, and "objective" knowledge as a triad (Hutchinson, p. 26).
43. Hearnshaw, pp. 284, 286–288.
44. Koestler, pp. 34, 70–71.
45. Palmer, *Does the Center Hold?* pp. 36–37, 379.
46. Although scientists like Premack and Gardner have trained chimpanzees to communicate in sign language, their achievement falls short of human language acquisition, which is spontaneous (Hearnshaw, pp. 261–262.)
47. Hearnshaw, pp. 270–271, 282–284, 287–289.
48. Linguistic bewitchment has habitually plagued the philosophy of mind and its intellectual progeny. Even Plato fell under the spell of words, but modern philosophers in particular have been seduced by their false potential. The critical seductions occurred in the eighteenth century, when Vico made the overblown claim that language determines all the properties of thought and Berkeley dubbed language as the glue holding together all ideational reality. In the 1850s, de Saussure formally dedicated himself to a specialized study of language by creating the discipline of philology. By 1950, researchers were diligently applying tools from information theory, particularly with regard to redundancy and noise, to language. These developments induced even skeptics like Skinner to accept language as a subject of singularly crucial psychological concern. With language then fully in the limelight, attempts at linguistic simulations on machines sprang up through programs such as SHIRDLU and proposals that consciousness itself is an encoded language (Hearnshaw, pp. 265–267, 271, 276, 286–289, 294; Oldroyd, p. 12; Palmer, *Does the Center Hold?* pp. 100, 104; Palmer, *Looking at Philosophy*, pp. 192–193).

49. Koestler, pp. 57, 226–227, 231–266.
50. Marcuse, *One-Dimensional Man*, p. xv.
51. Palmer, *Does the Center Hold?* pp. 308, 368.
52. Palmer, *Looking at Philosophy*, pp. 293–294.
53. Priest, pp. 57–58, 62–63.
54. Jonathan Turner, "Mead, George Herbert," in Kuper and Kuper, eds., *The Social Science Encyclopedia*, p. 508.
55. Schellenberg, pp. 38–62.
56. Priest, p. 35.
57. Flew, p. 145.
58. Losee, pp. 131–132.
59. Priest, pp. 37–43.
60. Collinson, pp. 145–150.
61. Flew, pp. 374–377.
62. "Wittgenstein, Ludwig Josef Johann" (no author given), in Gregory, ed., *The Oxford Companion*, p. 811.
63. Priest, pp. 56–64.
64. Flew, pp. 309–310.
65. T. R. Miles, "Ryle, Gilbert," in Gregory, ed., *The Oxford Companion*, pp. 691–692.
66. Palmer, *Does the Center Hold?* pp. 143–153.
67. Priest, pp. 35–64.
68. Albert Gilgen, "Skinner, Burrhus F., " in Kuper and Kuper, eds., *The Social Science Encyclopedia*, pp. 752–753.
69. Schellenberg, pp. 87–111.
70. Flanagan, pp. 99–103.
71. Oldroyd, p. 12.
72. Palmer, *Does the Center Hold?* pp. 104–105.
73. Palmer, *Looking at Philosophy*, pp. 192–193.
74. Gerald Grob, "Origins of DSM-I: A Study in Appearance and Reality," *American Journal of Psychiatry* 148:4 (April 1991), p. 421.
75. The psychiatrist's handling of violence in particular has depended on wider social contexts and demands. There are few reliable ways of predicting whether specific persons are prone to future violent behavior. Nevertheless, psychiatrists working as agents of society must often act in presumptive

haste in deciding whether to incarcerate potentially assaultive patients [Carl Sherman, "MDs Urged to Take Lead Role in Efforts to Reduce Violence," *Clinical Psychiatry News* (January 1993), p. 23; Tardiff, p. 496].

76. Eichelman, p. 491.
77. William Glazer, "Psychiatry and Medical Necessity," *Psychiatric Annals* 22:7 (July 1992), p. 366.
78. Calvin Pierce, "APA Ready to Launch Practice Guidelines Era," *Clinical Psychiatry News* 20:6 (June 1992), pp. 1, 22.
79. Measuring Psychiatry's Cost-Effectiveness: When a Dollar Saved Is Not a Dollar Earned, *Psychiatric News* (19 June 1922), p. 24.
80. Tardiff, pp. 493, 496, 498.
81. Hearnshaw, pp. 246–249.
82. Ibid., pp. 124, 129, 130, 134.
83. There also appeared at this time internationally oriented journals, including the *Zeitschrift für Psychologie und Physiologie der Sinnesorgane*, *Journal de Psychologie normal et pathologique*, *British Journal of Psychology*, and *L'Année Psychologique*.
84. Hearnshaw, pp. 134, 137–138.
85. Training under Wundt helped to influence Emil Kraepelin in favor of institutional settings and concrete experimental methods. Kraepelin also came to see mental illnesses as collective categories. His method of gathering statistical data according to epidemiologic principles at the turn of the century first created concepts of mental illnesses as reified entities. Alzheimer, Nissl, Brodmann, and the other members of Kraepelin's neuropsychiatric department spread his ideas throughout the universities of Europe. His clinical approaches eventually also took root across the Atlantic in the United States, where early acceptance of statistical, epidemiological approaches to research prompted the predecessor of the American Psychiatric Association to endorse "a uniform system to gather data on mental diseases and mental hospitals." Psychiatrists became even more prone to deal

with patients as "uniform" collective categories during their military experiences in World War II. Consequently, by the time the first *Diagnostic and Statistical Manual* (DSM-I) appeared in 1952, the committee responsible for its publication had embraced the use of standardized diagnostic categories. The committee's chairman stated that "accurate diagnosis is the keystone of appropriate treatment and competent prognosis" while downplaying concerns that standardized categories would jeopardize the understanding of individual patients. With the development of later DSM versions, particularly those in use since the 1970s, categorization and description have become paramount. Many alarmed practitioners have voiced the concern that these developments will completely remove from psychiatry's ken the individual patient's life history, his inner experiences and suffering, and their subjective impact. Symbolic, schematic excesses of disease taxonomy carry the danger of expanding to vaporize personal meaning completely, leaving the arbitrariness of semantic emptiness and vacuous protocols and routines. Hierarchical lumping of phenomena by DSM harks back to the most primitive kinds of thought, which merely pigeonhole phenomena instead of really explaining them. Past historical examples from protoscience include the arbitrary categories into which the ancients forced their physical constructs and the pre-Darwinian classes of plants and animals catalogued by Carolus Linneaus [Andreasen, *The Broken Brain*, p. 14; Jacob Bronowski, *The Common Sense of Science* (Cambridge: Harvard University Press, 1978), p. 50; Flanagan, pp. 76, 128; Grob, pp. 421–426, 427–430; George N. Raines, quoted in Grob, p. 430; Mitchell Wilson, "DSM-III and the Transformation of American Psychiatry: A History," *American Journal of Psychiatry* 150:3 (March 1993), pp. 399–410; Winson, p. 63; Zangwill, "Kraepelin" in Gregory, ed., *The Oxford Companion*, p. 414].

86. Hearnshaw, pp. 137–140, 141–143.
87. Ibid., pp. 271, 273–274.

88. "Big Brother May Soon Be Another Party to Every Drug Prescription Transaction," *Psychiatric News* (3 July 1992), pp. 4, 12.

89. "Measuring Psychiatry's Cost-Effectiveness," p. 24.

90. Roger Coleman, "Utilization Management and Quality Care," *Psychiatric Annals* 22:7 (July 1992), pp. 356–360.

91. Jan Fawcett, "Utilization Management—We Don't Have to Love It—We've Got to Learn About It," *Psychiatric Annals* 22:7 (July 1992), p. 354.

92. Daniel Moore, "Utilization Management and Outpatient Treatment," *Psychiatric Annals* 22:7 (July 1992), pp. 373–377.

93. "Psychotherapy Under the Knife," *U.S. News and World Report* (24 May 1993), p. 64.

94. Joyce Edward and Karen Shore, "The Trauma of Managed Mental Health Care," *New York Times* (15 February 1993), p. A14.

95. Janet Kamin, "When Managed Care Manages Psychotherapy," *New York Times* (13 May 1993), p. A22.

96. Elisabeth Rosenthal, "Insurers Second-Guess Doctors, Provoking Debate Over Savings," *The New York Times* (24 January 1993), pp. 1, 22.

97. "Big Brother," pp. 4, 12.

98. Fawcett, p. 354.

99. Glazer, pp. 363–365.

100. Moore, pp. 373–377.

101. Harold Alan Pincus and Theodora Fine, "The 'Anatomy' of Research Funding of Mental Illness and Addictive Disorders," *Archives of General Psychiatry* 49 (July 1992), p. 578.

102. "Measuring Psychiatry's Cost-Effectiveness," p. 24.

103. Eccles, pp. 351–353.

104. Flanagan, pp. 201, 203–206.

105. Erich Fromm, *The Sane Society* (New York: Henry Holt and Company, 1955), p. 122.

106. Goodman, p. 560.

107. Eysenck, *Decline and Fall of the Freudian Empire*, p. 204.

108. Barrett, *Irrational Man*, p. 163.

109. Norman O. Brown, *Life Against Death* (Middletown: Wesleyan University Press, 1959), p. 253.
110. Flanagan, p. 215.
111. Freedman and van Nieuwenhuizen, pp. 132, 134.
112. Kerner, pp. 176–177.
113. Koestler, p. 228.
114. Kramer, pp. 442–447.
115. Palmer, *Does the Center Hold?* pp. 320–323, 476–477.
116. Palmer, *Looking at Philosophy*, pp. 293–294, 320–323.
117. Priest, p. 93.
118. Scruton, *Kant*, pp. 67–68.
119. Koestler, pp. 309–310.
120. Palmer, *Does the Center Hold?* pp. 458–460.
121. Palmer, *Looking at Philosophy*, pp. 238–243.
122. Henry Margenau, *The Nature of Physical Reality* (Woodbridge: Oxbow Press, 1977), pp. 427–447.
123. Flanagan, p. 87.
124. Bronowski, *Magic, Science, and Civilization*, p. 17.
125. Marcuse, *One-Dimensional Man*, p. 164.
126. Palmer, *Does the Center Hold?* pp. 476–477.
127. Marcuse, *One-Dimensional Man*, p. 164.
128. Brown, p. 279.
129. Chester Finn, "The Campus: 'An Island of Repression in a Sea of Freedom,'" *Commentary* (September 1989), pp. 18–20, 22.
130. Koestler, pp. 226–227, 231–266.
131. Doris Lessing, "Language and the Lunatic Fringe," *New York Times* (26 June 1992), p. A27.
132. Camille Paglia, "Ninnies, Pedants, Tyrants, and Other Academics," *New York Times Book Review* (5 May 1991), pp. 1, 29.
133. Palmer, *Does the Center Hold?* p. 40.
134. Harold Morowitz, *Mayonnaise and the Origin of Life* (New York: Berkeley, 1985), pp. 110–111.
135. Jacques Barzun, *Darwin, Marx, Wagner* (Garden City: Doubleday, 1958), p. 338.
136. Genova, p. 19.

137. Sherman, p. 23.

138. Genova, p. 19.

139. R. Coleman, p. 360.

140. Glazer, pp. 362–366.

141. Moore, pp. 373–377.

142. Erica Goode and Betsy Wagner, "Does Psychotherapy Work?" *U.S. News and World Report* (24 May 1993), pp. 56–65.

143. Janice Krupnick and Harold Alan Pincus, "The Cost-Effectiveness of Psychotherapy: A Plan for Research," *American Journal of Psychiatry* 149:10 (October 1992), pp. 1295–1305.

144. Stephen Slatkin, "Short-Term Treatment, Better Results: IS-TDP," *Psychiatric Times* (March 1993), pp. 23–27.

145. R. Coleman, pp. 356–360.

146. Fawcett p. 354.

147. Genova, p. 19.

148. Glazer, pp. 363–364, 366.

149. Moore, p. 376.

150. Pierce, pp. 1, 22.

151. "Measuring Psychiatry's Cost-Effectiveness," p. 24.

152. Ernest Becker, *The Denial of Death* (New York: Macmillan, 1973), pp. 72–73.

153. Flanagan, p. 16.

154. Winson, pp. 135–136.

155. Flanagan, pp. 41, 106.

156. Koestler, pp. 3, 15, 130.

157. Fodor, p. 122.

158. Arnold Relman, "What Market Values Are Doing To Medicine," *Atlantic Monthly* (March 1992), p. 101.

159. Palmer, *Does the Center Hold?* pp. 402–403.

160. Arendt, pp. 7, 11.

161. Capra, pp. 381–383.

162. Ibid., pp. 370–371.

163. Alastair Bruce and David Wallace, "Critical Point Phenomena: Universal Physics at Large Length Scales," in *The New Physics*, ed. P. Davies (Cambridge: Cambridge University Press, 1989), pp. 236–267.

164. Kenneth Wilson, "Problems in Physics with Many Scales of Length," *Scientific American* 241 (August 1979), pp. 158–179.
165. E. T. Bell, pp. 340–361.
166. Bernstein and Phillips, pp. 126–127.
167. Freedman and van Nieuwenhuizen, pp. 132, 137.
168. Howard Georgi, "A Unified Theory of Elementary Particles and Forces," *Scientific American* 244 (April 1981), pp. 48–49.
169. R. I. G. Hughes, "Quantum Logic," *Scientific American* 245 (Oct 1981), pp. 205, 211.
170. Kramer, pp. 304–307, 350.
171. Ernst Sondheimer and Alan Rogerson, *Numbers and Infinity* (Cambridge: Cambridge University Press, 1981), pp. 69–85.
172. Singh, pp. 85–87.
173. David Spergel and Neil Turok, "Textures and Cosmic Structure," *Scientific American* 266 (March 1992), pp. 55, 57–58.
174. t'Hooft, pp. 118, 122.
175. Steven Weinberg, "Unified Theories of Elementary Particle Interaction," *Scientific American* 231 (July 1974), p. 54.

Chapter 10

1. Brown, pp. 236, 240, 245, 257–264, 271–272, 282.
2. Palmer, *Does the Center Hold?* pp. 397–398.
3. Palmer, *Looking at Philosophy*, p. 301.
4. Glazer, p. 363.
5. Moore, pp. 373–377.
6. Heilbroner, *The Wordly Philosophers* (New York: Simon and Schuster, 1972), p. 24.
7. Capra, p. 194.
8. Heilbroner, *The Wordly Philosophers*, pp. 26–27.
9. Capra, p. 194.
10. Heilbroner, *The Wordly Philosophers*, p. 34.
11. Ibid., p. 31.
12. Capra, p. 197.
13. Flew, pp. 327–328.

14. A. S. Skinner, "Smith, Adam," in Kuper and Kuper, eds., *The Social Science Encyclopedia*, pp. 756–758.
15. Heilbroner, *The Wordly Philosophers*, pp. 66, 69.
16. Ibid., p. 294.
17. Capra, p. 199.
18. Ibid., pp. 188–189, 213.
19. Heilbroner, *The Wordly Philosophers*, pp. 19, 55–57.
20. Ibid., p. 70.
21. Capra, p. 199.
22. Heilbroner, *The Wordly Philosophers*, pp. 91, 95, 97.
23. Charles Mann, "How Many is Too Many?" *Atlantic Monthly* (February 1993), pp. 47–67.
24. Heilbroner, *The Wordly Philosophers*, p. 256.
25. Ibid., p. 111.
26. Capra, pp. 203–204.
27. Heilbroner, *The Wordly Philosophers*, pp. 126–128.
28. Ibid., p. 202.
29. Capra, p. 209.
30. Heilbroner, *The Wordly Philosophers*, p. 203.
31. Ibid., pp. 190–191.
32. Ibid., p. 256.
33. Ibid., pp. 259–260, 264–265.
34. Ibid., p. 268.
35. Capra, pp. 190–191, 225–226.
36. Ibid., pp. 189, 196.
37. Flew, p. 327.
38. Harvey Goldman, *Max Weber and Thomas Mann* (Berkeley: University of California Press, 1988), pp. 18–51.
39. Stephen Kalberg, "Weber, Max," in Kuper and Kuper, eds., *The Social Science Encyclopedia*, pp. 892–896.
40. David Held, *Introduction to Critical Theory* (Berkeley: University of California Press, 1980), pp. 64–66.
41. John Whitworth, "Veblen, Thorstein Bunde," in Kuper and Kuper, eds., *The Social Science Encyclopedia*, pp. 880–881.
42. Heilbroner, *The Wordly Philosophers*, pp. 223–226.
43. Capra, p. 215.

44. Heilbroner, *The Wordly Philosophers*, pp. 225, 230.
45. Kurt Rothschild, "Schumpeter, Joseph Alois," in Kuper and Kuper, eds., *The Social Science Encyclopedia*, pp. 731–732.
46. Heilbroner, *The Wordly Philosophers*, pp. 235, 237–238.
47. Ibid., pp. 309–310.
48. Capra, pp. 212, 220–221, 223, 227–228.
49. David McLelland, "Marx, Karl Heinrich," in Kuper and Kuper, eds., *The Social Science Encyclopedia*, pp. 493–495.
50. Collinson, pp. 110–111.
51. Peter Singer, *Marx* (Oxford: Oxford University Press, 1980), pp. 1–10.
52. Heilbroner, *Marxism: For and Against* (New York: Norton, 1980), p. 143.
53. Ibid., pp. 15–18.
54. Ibid., p. 80.
55. Hearnshaw, p. 176.
56. Capra, pp. 208–209.
57. Robert Tucker, *Philosophy and Myth in Karl Marx* (London: Cambridge University Press, 1972), pp. 141–143.
58. Heilbroner, *Marxism*, p. 63.
59. Ibid., p. 68.
60. Capra, pp. 206–207.
61. Heilbroner, *Marxism*, p. 72.
62. Ibid., pp. 95, 102–103, 148.
63. Ibid., pp. 96–97.
64. Ibid., pp. 105–106.
65. Ibid., pp. 110, 121.
66. Ibid., pp. 116, 135.
67. R. Tucker, pp. 137, 139, 145–149, 158.
68. Ibid., pp. 138–141, 158.
69. Capra, pp. 230–231.
70. Heilbroner, *Marxism*, pp. 117, 140–141, 151, 153–154, 158.
71. R. Tucker, p. 141.
72. Heilbroner, *Marxism*, pp. 135, 168.
73. Held, pp. 29–39, 112–115, 121–126.
74. Hampden-Turner, *Maps of the Mind*, pp. 186–189.

75. Douglas Kellner, "Frankfurt School," in Kuper and Kuper, eds., *The Social Science Encyclopedia*, pp. 311–313.
76. Robert M. Young, "Publisher's Foreword," In Marcuse, *Negations*, p. viii.
77. Kellner, "Marcuse, Herbert," in Kuper and Kuper, eds., *The Social Science Encyclopedia*, p. 483.
78. Elements extrinsic to quaternions might partially repress the threefold invariance of self-identities by acting in a manner analogous to the so-called Higgs field of particle physics [P. Davies and J. Brown, *Superstrings* (Cambridge: Cambridge University Press, 1988), p. 55; Sondheimer and Rogerson, pp. 69–85].
79. Davies and Brown, pp. 54–55.
80. John Allen Paulos, "Fearful Symmetry," *New York Times Book Review* (28 June 1992), p. 11.
81. Georgi, pp. 58–59.
82. This pattern of splitting and sparing may occur insofar as the symmetry-breaking form of epistemic torsion is connected with mappings between a field's local and nonlocal features. Alternative deformities of two specific kinds should result from such mappings. These deformities could create an antipodal schism in the topology of *Dasein* that preserves the twofold subsymmetry between collective and fragmented self-distortions, yet splits away the soma (Bernstein and Phillips, pp. 128, 130; Manin, pp. 81–84; Peat, pp. 147, 155, 176–180; Penrose, "The Geometry of the Universe," pp. 85–89, 91, 122–123).
83. Marcuse, *One-Dimensional Man*, pp. xiv, 154.
84. Flanagan, pp. xiii, 163.
85. Huston Smith, *The Religions of Man* (New York: Harper & Row, 1986), p. 26.
86. Barrett, *The Death of The Soul*, p. 41.
87. Flanagan, pp. 225, 227–232, 254–256.
88. Foucault, pp. 23–24, 52, 63, 84, 88.
89. Hampden-Turner, pp. 60–63.
90. Kerner, p. 197.

91. Ladd, p. 59.
92. Palmer, *Does the Center Hold?* p. 408.
93. Marcuse, *One-Dimensional Man*, pp. 145–146, 154, 168.
94. Kerner, p. 191.
95. Capra, p. 199.
96. Brown, p. 253.
97. Freedman and van Nieuwenhuizen, pp. 132, 134.
98. Heilbroner, *Marxism*, pp. 96–100.
99. Kerner, pp. 176–177.
100. Kramer, pp. 442–447.
101. Priest, p. 93.
102. According to Marcuse, styles of logic used by humans throughout history have varied in accordance with the demands of different cultures at different times. Logical styles have included the Greek syllogism, transcendental and dialectical reasoning, and formal symbolism. Mathematical logic is the latest among these modes of thought (Marcuse, *One-Dimensional Man*, pp. 167–168).
103. Ibid., p. 169.
104. Ibid., p. 144.
105. Ibid., p. 157.
106. Brown, pp. 131, 279, 388.
107. Capra, pp. 197, 199.
108. Relman, pp. 100, 102.
109. Ibid., pp. 101, 102, 105.
110. Ibid., p. 102.
111. Pincus and Fine, p. 573.
112. Capra, p. 211.
113. Brown, pp. 29, 31, 79, 195, 245, 257–258, 282, 288, 293.
114. Capra, pp. 190–191, 215, 229–230.
115. Foucault, p. 68.
116. Marcuse, *One-Dimensional Man*, pp. 145–146.
117. Palmer, *Does the Center Hold?* pp. 301–304, 468–471, 278.
118. Foucault, p. 68.
119. Hearnshaw, p. 247.
120. Moore, pp. 373–376.

121. Richard Karel, "Congress Gets Earful on Psych Hospitals," *Psychiatric News* (19 June 1992), p. 26.
122. Relman, pp. 100–106.
123. Karel, pp. 1, 26.
124. Foucault, pp. 68, 76–77.
125. Capra, p. 189.
126. Ibid., p. 191.
127. Marcuse, *One-Dimensional Man*, pp. 154, 162–163.
128. Ibid., pp. xii–xiii, 145–146.
129. Ibid., p. 169.
130. Bertram Bernstein, "What Will Protect Us from Managed Care?" *New York Times* (3 August 1993), p. A16.
131. R. Coleman, pp. 356–360, 362.
132. Edward and Shore, p. A14.
133. Fawcett, p. 354.
134. William Glazer, "Overview of Utilization Management," *Psychiatric Annals* 22:7 (July 1992), p. 355.
135. Glazer, pp. 362, 366.
136. David Himmelstein and Steffie Woolhandler, "Clinton Plan Will Restrict Health Care Choice," *New York Times* (26 September 1993), p. E14.
137. Kamin, p. A22.
138. "Measuring Psychiatry's Cost-Effectiveness," p. 24.
139. Moore, pp. 373–375.
140. Pierce, pp. 1, 22.
141. "Psychotherapy Under the Knife," p. 64.
142. Rosenthal, pp. 1, 22.
143. Palmer, *Does the Center Hold?* pp. 313–315, 400–401.
144. Palmer, *Looking at Philosophy*, pp. 298–299, 302.
145. Harold Varmus and Marc Kirschner, "Don't Undermine Basic Research," *New York Times* (29 September 1992), p. A27.
146. Flanagan, pp. 112–113, 165–166.
147. Palmer, *Does the Center Hold?* pp. 291–292.
148. Leon Lederman, "Science and the Bottom Line," *New York Times* (16 September 1993), p. A23.
149. Palmer, *Looking at Philosophy*, pp. 238–243.

150. Pincus and Fine, pp. 573–579.
151. Even further centralization is now under way, as the NIMH, NIDA, and NIAAA lose their autonomy and begin reporting directly to the overall management of the NIH. This will leave the top of the NIH controlling not only NIMH, NIDA, and NIAAA money but also psychiatrically earmarked funds from the National Institute of Neurological Disorders and Stroke, the National Institute on Aging, the National Institute on Child Health and Human Development, the National Heart, Lung and Blood Institute, and the National Institute on Diabetes and Digestive and Kidney Diseases ["ADAMHA Reorganization Plan Approved by President Bush," *Psychiatric Times* (7 August 1992), pp. 1, 24; Pincus and Fine, p. 579].
152. Pincus and Fine, p. 579.
153. Ibid., pp. 576, 579.
154. For example, in 1988, the Social Security Administration supported work on disability, the Health Care Finance Administration aided development of psychiatric diagnostic nosology related to reimbursement, the Department of Education sponsored studies on learning disabilities and rehabilitation, the Department of Justice funded research on substance abuse and violence, and the Defense Department and NASA maintained involvement with investigations related to crew behavior and circadian rhythms (Pincus and Fine, p. 577).
155. Pincus and Fine, p. 578.
156. Grob, p. 421.
157. Brown, pp. 260–261.
158. Palmer, *Does the Center Hold?* pp. 413, 461.
159. Palmer, *Looking at Philosophy*, p. 278.
160. The process of medical education encourages power-seeking behavior among physicians. Only the most competitive among applicants are selected for admission to medical school. During clinical training, medical students, interns, and residents are often pitted against their colleagues and

encouraged to "attack" disease processes aggressively. They are frequently discouraged from attending to their own spiritual health in an environment that emphasizes abusively long work hours and no room for personal development or private life.

161. Capra, pp. 147–148.
162. Ibid., 158–163.
163. The will to hierarchical dominance and elitism has an especially strong hold on academia. Some scholars see themselves as an elite group and appropriate language as an instrument of power, imposing explicit standards of linguistic correctness on those attempting to gain entry into their circle (Finn, pp. 17, 19–20; Lessing, p. A27; Paglia, p. 33).
164. Capra, p. 143.
165. Henry Pinsker, quoted in Mitchell Wilson, "DSM-III and the Transformation of American Psychiatry: A History," p. 405.
166. Capra, pp. 249–252.
167. Patrick Cody, "Numerous Drug Ads in Journals Judged Misleading, Inaccurate," *Psychiatric News* (21 August 1992), pp. 1, 19.
168. Glenn Miller, "Insanity Standards," *Psychiatric Annals* 22:12 (December 1992), pp. 626–631.
169. Restak, "See No Evil," pp. 16–21.
170. Tardiff, pp. 496–497.
171. Graham Locke, "Foucault, Michel," in Kuper and Kuper, eds., *The Social Science Encyclopedia*, pp. 310–311.
172. Nehamas, "Subject and Abject," *The New Republic* (15 February 1993), pp. 27–36.
173. David Shumway, *Michel Foucault* (Charlottesville: University Press of Virginia, 1989), chronology.
174. Locke, pp. 310–311.
175. Nehamas, pp. 30–31.
176. Daniel Bell, *The Cultural Contradictions of Capitalism* (New York: Basic Books, 1978), p. 34.
177. Foucault, pp. 63, 68.
178. Locke, pp. 310–311.

179. Mark Philip, "Foucault," in Skinner, ed., *The Return of Grand Theory in the Human Sciences*, pp. 63–81.
180. Shumway, pp. 27–45.
181. Marcuse, *One-Dimensional Man*, p. xv.
182. Jay Greenberg and Stephen Mitchell, *Object Relations in Psychoanalytic Theory* (Cambridge: Harvard University Press, 1983), p. 167.
183. Flanagan, p. 81.
184. Foucault, p. 46.
185. Palmer, *Does the Center Hold?* pp. 212–213, 402.
186. Davies and Brown, p. 57.

Chapter 11

1. S. Cooper, p. 272.
2. "Don't Replace Psychotherapy With a Pill, Experts Remind Public-Sector Psychiatrists," p. 13.
3. Glen Gabbard, "Psychodynamic Psychiatry in the 'Decade of the Brain,'" *American Journal of Psychiatry* 149:8 (August 1992), p. 996.
4. Capra, p. 368.
5. S. Cooper, p. 272.
6. Sigmund Freud, *An Autobiographical Study*, trans. James Strachey (New York: Norton, 1963), pp. 11–126.
7. Hearnshaw, pp. 156–165.
8. George Pollack, "Freud, Sigmund," in Kuper and Kuper, eds., *The Social Science Encyclopedia*, pp. 317–320.
9. Schellenberg, pp. 11–37.
10. O. L. Zangwill, "Freud, Sigmund," in Gregory, ed., *The Oxford Companion*, pp. 268–270.
11. Eysenck, pp. 201, 206.
12. Hearnshaw, p. 231.
13. Peter Medawar, *Pluto's Republic* (Oxford: Oxford University Press, 1982), pp. 62–72.
14. David Sachs, "In Fairness to Freud: A Critical Notice of The

Foundations of Psychoanalysis, by Adolf Grunbaum," in *The Cambridge Companion to Freud*, ed. Jerome Neu (Cambridge: Cambridge University Press, 1991), pp. 310, 312–313, 315–316, 332.

15. Winson, pp. 144, 146, 151–153.
16. Sachs, pp. 312, 313, 317, 319, 325, 327–328.
17. Winson, p. 135–136, 150.
18. Flanagan, p. 16.
19. Ibid.
20. Arnold Cooper, "Will Neurobiology Influence Psychoanalysis?" *American Journal of Psychiatry* 142: 12 (December 1985), pp. 1397–1398.
21. Gabbard, p. 994.
22. A. Cooper, p. 1396.
23. Winson, p. 66.
24. Sachs, p. 317.
25. Freud, *An Autobiographical Study*, pp. 25–26.
26. Frattaroli, p. 73.
27. Rieff, *Freud: The Mind of the Moralist*, quoted in Eysenck, p. 196.
28. Flanagan, pp. 63, 65, 81.
29. Gabbard, pp. 991, 993.
30. A. Cooper, p. 1395.
31. Ibid.
32. Flanagan, pp. 63, 65, 81.
33. Gabbard, p. 991.
34. Bronowski, *A Sense of the Future*, pp. 67–68.
35. Winson, pp. 85, 110–111.
36. Gabbard, p. 993.
37. Frattaroli, p. 77.
38. George Goethals, "Sullivan, Harry Stack," in Kuper and Kuper, eds., *The Social Science Encyclopedia*, pp. 841–842.
39. Greenberg and Mitchell, p. 85.
40. Jean Shinoda Bolen, "Jung, Carl Gustav," in Kuper and Kuper, eds., *The Social Science Encyclopedia*, pp. 420–421.
41. Capra, pp. 362–363.

42. D. A. G. Cook, "Jung, Carl Gustav," in Gregory, ed., *The Oxford Companion*, pp. 403–405.
43. Hearnshaw, p. 166.
44. A. Cooper, p. 1397.
45. Gabbard, p. 996.
46. A. Cooper, p. 1397.
47. Capra, p. 185.
48. Johnson-Laird, pp. 20–21.
49. Kaplan and Sadock, pp. 147–149.
50. Schellenberg, p. 63.
51. Jacques Barzun, *A Stroll with William James* (New York: Harper & Row, 1983), pp. 6–33.
52. Collinson, pp. 116–119.
53. Flew, p. 184.
54. Hearnshaw, pp. 143–148.
55. Ian Hunter, "James, William," in Gregory, ed., *The Oxford Companion*, pp. 395–397.
56. Russell, pp. 811–818.
57. H. S. Thayer, "James, William," in Kuper and Kuper, eds., *The Social Science Encyclopedia*, pp. 417–418.
58. Hearnshaw, pp. 291–292.
59. Capra, p. 233.
60. Morowitz, *Mayonnaise and the Origin of Life*, p. 164.
61. Capra, pp. 117–118.
62. Schrödinger, *My View of the World*, pp. 8–9.
63. John Stuart Mill, *Principles of Political Economy*, book 3, chapter 7, section 5, quoted in Berlin, *The Crooked Timber of Humanity* (New York: Random House, 1992), p. 90.
64. Bronowski, *A Sense of the Future*, p. 69.
65. Bronowski, *The Identity of Man*, pp. 81–82, 114.
66. Havel, "The End of the Modern Era," p. E15.
67. Francois Jacob, *The Logic of Life* (New York: Pantheon, 1973), pp. 320–321.
68. Morowitz, *Mayonnaise and the Origin of Life*, pp. 110–111.
69. Jacob Bronowski, *The Ascent of Man* (London: Futura, 1973), p. 266.

70. Barrett, *Irrational Man*, pp. 225–227.
71. Frattaroli, p. 74.
72. Eysenck, p. 198, 201.
73. Winson, p. 155.
74. Eysenck, p. 205.
75. Winson, p. 149.
76. Collinson, pp. 107–110.
77. Flew, pp. 193–194.
78. "Kierkegaard, Soren Aaby" (no author given), in Gregory, ed., *The Oxford Companion*, pp. 268–270.
79. Barrett, *Irrational Man*, pp. 151, 165, 170–171.
80. Hearnshaw, pp. 233–234, 237.
81. Palmer, *Looking at Philosophy*, p. 361.
82. Scruton, *Kant*, pp. 59, 66, 76–77.
83. Christoph Mundt, "Images in Psychiatry: Karl Jaspers," *American Journal of Psychiatry* 150:8 (August 1993), pp. 1244–1245.
84. A. Cooper, p. 1396.
85. Ibid., p. 1397.
86. Ibid.
87. Gabbard, pp. 995–996.
88. Becker, pp. 69–70, 92.
89. Gabbard, pp. 995–996.
90. Frattaroli, p. 74.
91. Hearnshaw, p. 137.
92. Palmer, *Does the Center Hold?* p. 36.
93. Becker, pp. 86–88, 92.
94. Jose Ortega y Gasset, *The Revolt of the Masses*, authorized anonymous translation from the Spanish (New York: Norton, 1932), p. 170.
95. Freud, "Psychoanalysis and Telepathy," quoted in Capra, p. 180.
96. Becker, pp. 69–70, 92.
97. Winson, pp. 134–135.
98. Frattaroli, p. 73.
99. Winson, pp. 134–135.

100. Philip Rieff, *Freud: The Mind of the Moralist* (Chicago: University of Chicago Press, 1979), p. 13.
101. Winson, pp. 134–135.
102. Becker, p. 68.
103. Ibid., p. 87.
104. Havel, p. E15.
105. Palmer, *Does the Center Hold?* pp. 247–249.
106. Greenberg and Mitchell, p. 110.
107. i.e., "genital."
108. i.e., "anal."
109. i.e., "oral."
110. Barrett, *The Death of The Soul*, p. 120.
111. Barrett, *Irrational Man*, p. 229.
112. Brown, pp. 11–12, 15, 92–93, 101–109, 236, 240, 245, 257–264, 271–275, 277–278, 282–283, 297.
113. Flanagan, pp. 166–168.
114. Greenberg and Mitchell, pp. 108–110.
115. Koestler, pp. 300–302, 312.
116. Palmer, *Looking at Philosophy*, pp. 225–226.
117. Hearnshaw, pp. 232–234, 243.
118. Koestler, pp. 86–94.
119. Flanagan, pp. 69–70.
120. Frattaroli, p. 74.
121. Volkow and Tancredi, "Biological Correlates," pp. 441–442.
122. Brown, pp. 28, 60.
123. Koestler, pp. 121, 140–142, 163–169, 179–180.
124. Palmer, *Does the Center Hold?* pp. 247–249, 466–467.
125. Koestler, pp. 205–219.
126. Flanagan, pp. 157–159, 168, 171.
127. Barrett, *Irrational Man*, pp. 168–169.
128. Palmer, *Does the Center Hold?* pp. 397–398.
129. Barrett, *Irrational Man*, p. 172.
130. A. Cooper, p. 1401.
131. Ibid., pp. 1395, 1396.
132. Kandel, pp. 1028–1029.
133. A. Cooper, pp. 1396, 1402.

134. Ibid., p. 1397.

135. Ibid., p. 1396.

136. Gabbard, p. 992.

137. Winson, pp. 173, 220.

138. Gabbard, p. 996.

139. Gerald Klerman, "Depression and Related Disorders of Mood (Affective Disorders)," in Nicholi, ed., *The New Harvard Guide*, pp. 329–332, 334.

140. Meissner, p. 467.

141. Tomb, p. 178.

142. Kaplan and Sadock, p. 269.

143. Meissner, p. 463.

144. Tomb, pp. 28, 46, 154, 178.

145. Tsuang *et al.*, pp. 276–277.

146. Gabbard, p. 991, 993.

147. Ibid., pp. 994–995.

148. Kaplan and Sadock, pp. 303, 329.

149. Meissner, p. 467.

150. John C. Nemiah, "Psychoneurotic Disorders," in Nicholi, ed., *The New Harvard Guide*, pp. 238, 244–245, 303.

151. Tomb, p. 154.

152. Gabbard, pp. 991, 993–995.

153. Anna M. Spielvogel, M.D., director of residency training at San Francisco General Hospital, quoted in "Don't Replace Psychotherapy With a Pill," p. 13.

154. Gabbard, pp. 992, 996.

155. Ibid., p. 991.

156. Gabbard *et al.*, p. 21.

157. Gabbard, pp. 993, 995.

158. Flanagan, p. 178.

159. Marcuse, *Negations*, pp. 58–60.

160. Priest, pp. 198–199, 207.

161. Winson, p. 117.

162. Ibid.

163. Frattaroli, p. 77.

164. The string theories of modern particle physics may provide a

useful analogy here. Two-vectored play in the economic symmetry between collective and fragmented self-distortions may repress individual selfhood by twisting and squeezing the split-off curvature of somatic self-identity into a separate, one-dimensional straightjacket. This structure could be analogous to a subatomic "string." Stringlike confinement of noneconomic self-relations within the individual domain would condense and fuse subsumed gauge field intentionalities, paradoxically mixing together intentional meanings even if they were mutually contradictory from an economic point of view. This might feed our culture's perception of noneconomic behavior as an irrational mental state with morbidly regressive dynamics [Brown, pp. 25–27, 88, 111–112, 116–117, 257–258, 288; Flanagan, p. 354; Freedman and van Nieuwenhuizen, pp. 128, 132, 134; Susan James, "Louis Althusser," in Skinner, ed., *The Return of Grand Theory*, p. 148; Koestler, pp. 192–194, 218, 228–229, 246–247; Yoichiro Nambu, "The Confinement of Quarks," *Scientific American* 235 (November 1976), pp. 57–60; Palmer, *Does the Center Hold?* pp. 212–213, 402].

165. Capra, pp. 368–369.
166. A structure resembling the "fiber bundles" of modern physics could impose local symmetry properties on torsional nonlocality and restore expression of the hidden symmetry among all three vectors of self-scale. The relevant route would involve analogies to so-called "cohomological" transformations originating in symmetry breakage defects. Testing of the validity of this approach might involve a backward mapping from the final "fiber bundle" into the original, globally symmetric model of functionalism to obtain an "objective" readout in real numbers (Georgi, pp. 61, 63; Peat, pp. 176–180, 183–185, 217–223, 267–268; Spergel and Turok, pp. 55, 57–58).

Bibliography

"ADAMHA Reorganization Plan Approved by President Bush," *The Psychiatric Times* (7 August 1992), pp. 1, 24.

Adams, Raymond, and Maurice Victor, *Principles of Neurology* (New York: McGraw-Hill, 1977), 1041 pp.

Aleksandrov, A. D., A. N. Kolmogorov, and M. A. Lavrent'ev, *Mathematics*, Volume 3 (Cambridge: MIT Press, 1963), 372 pp.

Allen, Garland, *Life Sciences in the Twentieth Century* (Cambridge: Cambridge University Press, 1978), 257 pp.

American Psychiatric Association, *Biographical Directory* (Washington: American Psychiatric Association, 1989), 1943 pp.

Andreasen, Nancy, *The Broken Brain* (New York: Harper & Row, 1984), 278 pp.

Andreasen, Nancy, ed., *Brain Imaging: Applications in Psychiatry* (Washington: American Psychiatric Press, 1989), 384 pp.

Andreasen, Nancy, Gregg Cohen, Greg Harris, Ted Cizaldo, Jussi Parkkinen, Karim Rezai, and Victor Swayze, "Image Processing for the Study of Brain Structure and Function: Problems and Programs," *Journal of Neuropsychiatry* 4:2 (Spring 1992), pp. 125–133.

Arendt, Hannah, *The Life of the Mind* (New York: Harcourt Brace Jovanovich, 1978), 283 pp.

Aronowitz, Stanley, *Science as Power* (Minneapolis: University of Minnesota Press, 1988), 384 pp.

Ayd, Frank, "Novel Antipsychotics, Antidepressants Surveyed in S.F.," *Psychiatric Times* (August 1993), pp. 7–8.

Ayer, A. J., *Philosophy in the Twentieth Century* (New York: Vintage, 1982), 283 pp.

Baldessarini, Ross, *Chemotherapy in Psychiatry* (Cambridge: Harvard University Press, 1985), 354 pp.

Barr, Linda, "Serotonin in Obsessive–Compulsive Disorder," *Psychiatric Times* (July 1993), pp. 24–25.

Barrett, William, *The Death of the Soul* (Garden City, NY: Doubleday, 1986), 173 pp.

Barrett, William, *The Illusion of Technique* (Garden City, NY: Anchor, 1976), 392 pp.

Barrett, William, *Irrational Man* (New York: Doubleday, 1958), 314 pp.

Barzun, Jacques, *Darwin, Marx, Wagner* (Garden City, NY: Doubleday, 1958), 373 pp.

Barzun, Jacques, *A Stroll with William James* (New York: Harper & Row, 1983), 344 pp.

Bateson, Gregory, *Mind and Nature* (New York: Bantam, 1979), 255 pp.

Beakley, Brian, and Peter Ludlow, eds., *The Philosophy of Mind* (Cambridge: MIT Press, 1992), 433 pp.

Becker, Ernest, *The Denial of Death* (New York: Macmillan, 1973), 314 pp.

Bell, Daniel, *The Cultural Contradictions of Capitalism* (New York: Basic Books, 1978), 301 pp.

Bell, E. T., *Men of Mathematics* (New York: Simon & Schuster, 1965), 895 pp.

Benacerraf, Paul, and Hillary Putnam, eds., *Philosophy of Mathematics* (Cambridge: Cambridge University Press, 1964), 600 pp.

Bennett, Charles, Gilles Brassard, and Artur K. Ekert, "Quantum Cryptography," *Scientific American* 267 (October 1992), pp. 50–57.

Berlin, Isaiah, *The Crooked Timber of Humanity* (New York: Random House, 1992), 278 pp.

Bernstein, Bertram, "What Will Protect Us from Managed Care?" *The New York Times* (3 August 1993), p. A16.

Bernstein, Herbert, and Anthony Phillips, "Fiber Bundles and Quantum Theory," *Scientific American* 245 (July 1981), pp. 123–137.

Bernstein, Jeremy, *The Analytical Engine* (New York: William Morrow, 1981), 131 pp.

Bettelheim, Bruno, *Freud and Man's Soul* (New York: Vintage, 1982), 112 pp.

"Big Brother May Soon Be Another Party to Every Drug Prescription Transaction," *Psychiatric News* (3 July 1992), pp. 4, 12.

Blakemore, Colin, and Susan Greenfield, eds., *Mindwaves* (Oxford: Basil Blackwell, 1987), 525 pp.

Blakeslee, Sandra, "Scanner Pinpoints Site of Thought as Brain Sees or Speaks," *The New York Times* (1 June 1993), pp. C1, C3.

Blakeslee, Sandra, "Scientists Unraveling Chemistry of Dreams," *The New York Times* (7 January 1992), pp. C1, C10.

Bloom, Allan, *The Closing of the American Mind* (New York: Simon & Schuster, 1987), 282 pp.

Bochner, Salomon, *The Role of Mathematics in the Physical Sciences* (Princeton: Princeton University Press, 1966), 386 pp.

Bohm, David, *Wholeness and the Implicate Order* (London: Ark, 1980), 220 pp.

Boyer, Carl, *A History of Mathematics* (Princeton: Princeton University Press, 1968), 717 pp.

Bracewell, Ronald, "The Fourier Transform," *Scientific American* 260 (June 1989), pp. 86–95.

Brandsetter, Robert W., Lois Brandsetter, Deanne Brandsetter, and Robert D. Brandsetter, "Artificial Neural Networks: One Step Too Far?," *New York State Journal of Medicine* 91:7 (July 1991), pp. 305–306.

Brazier, Mary, *Electrical Activity of the Nervous System* (Baltimore: Williams & Wilkins, 1977), 248 pp.

Brenner, Charles, *An Elementary Textbook of Psychoanalysis* (Garden City, NY: Anchor, 1973), 260 pp.

Briggs, John, and F. David Peat, *Looking Glass Universe* (New York: Simon & Schuster, 1984), 290 pp.

Bronowski, Jacob, *The Ascent of Man* (London: Futura, 1973), 287 pp.

Bronowski, Jacob, *The Common Sense of Science* (Cambridge: Harvard University Press, 1978), 150 pp.

Bronowski, Jacob, *The Identity of Man* (Garden City, NY: The Natural History Press, 1966), 145 pp.

Bronowski, Jacob, *Magic, Science, and Civilization* (New York: Columbia University Press, 1978), 88 pp.

Bronowski, Jacob, *The Origins of Knowledge and Imagination* (New Haven: Yale University Press, 1978), 144 pp.

Bronowski, Jacob, *A Sense of the Future* (Cambridge: MIT Press, 1977), 286 pp.

Browder, Felix, "Does Pure Mathematics Have a Relation to the Sciences?," *American Scientist* 64 (September–October 1976), pp. 542–549.

Brown, Norman O., *Life Against Death* (Middletown, CT: Wesleyan University Press, 1959), 366 pp.

Bunge, Mario, *Causality and Modern Science* (New York: Dover, 1979), 394 pp.

Callahan, J. J., "The Curvature of Space in a Finite Universe," *Scientific American* 235 (August 1976), pp. 90–100.

Calvin, William, *The Throwing Madonna* (New York: McGraw-Hill, 1983), 253 pp.

Campbell, Jeremy, *Grammatical Man* (New York: Simon & Schuster, 1982), 319 pp.

Canguilhem, Georges, *Ideology and Rationality in the History of the Life Sciences*, trans. Arthur Goldhammer (Cambridge: MIT Press, 1988), 160 pp.

Capra, Fritjof, *The Turning Point* (New York: Bantam, 1982), 464 pp.

Chaitin, Gregory, "Randomness and Mathematic Proof," *Scientific American* 232 (May 1975), pp. 47–52.

Chancer, Lynn, *Sadomasochism in Everyday Life* (New Brunswick, NJ: Rutgers University Press, 1992), 238 pp.

Changeux, Jean-Pierre, *Neuronal Man* (Oxford: Oxford University Press, 1985), 348 pp.

Cody, Patrick, "Numerous Drug Ads in Journals Judged Misleading, Inaccurate," *Psychiatric News* (21 August 1992), pp. 1, 19.

Cohen, Jonathan, and David Servan-Schreiber, "Introduction to Neural Network Models in Psychiatry," *Psychiatric Annals* 22:3 (March 1922), pp. 113–118.

Cohen, Jonathan, and David Servan-Schreiber, "A Neural Network Model of Disturbances in the Processing of Context in Schizophrenia," *Psychiatric Annals* 22:3 (March 1922), pp. 131–136.

Cohen, Paul, and Reuben Hersh, "Non-Cantorian Set Theory," *Scientific American* 217 (December 1967), pp. 104–116.

Coleman, Roger, "Utilization Management and Quality Care," *Psychiatric Annals* 22:7 (July 1992), pp. 356–361.

Collinson, Diane, *Fifty Major Philosophers* (London: Croom Helm, 1987), 170 pp.

Cooper, Arnold, "Will Neurobiology Influence Psychoanalysis?" *American Journal of Psychiatry* 142:12 (December 1985), pp. 1395–1402.

Cooper, Jack, Floyd Bloom, and Robert Roth, *The Biochemical Basis of Neuropharmacology* (New York: Oxford University Press, 1978), 327 pp.

Cooper, Steven, "Neuroscience in the Future of Psychiatry," *American Journal of Psychiatry* 145:2 (February 1988), pp. 272–273.

Crick, F. H. C., "Thinking About the Brain," in *The Brain*, eds. Gerard Piel *et al.* (San Francisco: W. H. Freeman, 1979), pp. 130–137.

Crossley, J. N., C. J. Ash, C. J. Brickhill, J. C. Stillwell, and N. H. Williams, *What Is Mathematical Logic?* (Oxford: Oxford University Press, 1972), 82 pp.

Cummings, Jeffrey, *Clinical Neuropsychiatry* (Orlando, FL: Grune & Stratton, 1985), 264 pp.

Cummings, Jeffrey, "Neurobiological Basis of Obsessive–Compulsive Disorder," *Psychiatric Times* (January 1993), p. 16.

D'Abro, A., *The Rise of the New Physics*, Volume 1 (New York: Dover, 1951), 426 pp.

Davies, P., *Space and Time in the Modern Universe* (Cambridge: Cambridge University Press, 1977), 232 pp.

Davies, P., ed., *The New Physics* (Cambridge: Cambridge University Press, 1989), 516 pp.

Davies, P., and Julian Brown, *Superstrings* (Cambridge: Cambridge University Press, 1988), 234 pp.

Davis, Martin, and Reuben Hersh, "Nonstandard Analysis," *Scientific American* 226 (June 1972), pp. 78–86.

Davis, Philip, and Reuben Hersh, *The Mathematical Experience* (Boston: Houghton Mifflin, 1981), 440 pp.

Davis, Philip, and David Park, eds., *No Way: The Nature of the Impossible* (New York: W. H. Freeman, 1987), 325 pp.

Delbruck, Max, *Mind from Matter?* (Palo Alto: Blackwell, 1986), 290 pp.

De Lecuona, Juan M., K. Sunny Joseph, Naveed Iqbal, and Gregory Asis, "Dopamine Hypothesis of Schizophrenia Revisited," *Psychiatric Annals* 23:4 (April 1993), pp. 179–185.

De Santillana, Giorgia, ed., *The Age of Adventure* (New York: Mentor, 1956), 283 pp.

Dominguez, Roberto, "Serotonergic Antidepressants and Their Efficacy in Obsessive Compulsive Disorder," *Journal of Clinical Psychiatry* 53:10 (October 1992 supplement), pp. 56–59.

"Don't Replace Psychotherapy with a Pill, Experts Remind Public-Sector Psychiatrists," *Psychiatric News* (3 July 1992), p. 13.

Drooker, Martin, and Robert Byck, "Physical Disorders Presenting as Psychiatric Illness: A New View," *Psychiatric Times* (July 1992), pp. 19–23.

Duncan, Ronald, and Miranda Weston-Smith, eds., *The Encyclopedia of Ignorance* (New York: Wallaby 1977), 443 pp.

Eccles, John, "A Critical Appraisal of Mind–Brain Theories," in *Cerebral Correlates of Conscious Experience*, eds., Buser and Rougeul-Buser (Oxford: Elsevier, 1978), pp. 347–355.

Edelson, Edward, "Scanning the Body Magnetic," *Science 83* (July–August 1983), pp. 60–65.

Edward, Joyce, and Karen Shore, "The Trauma of Managed Mental Health Care," *The New York Times* (15 February 1993), p. A14.

Eichelman, Burr, "Aggressive Behavior: From Laboratory to Clinic," *Archives of General Psychiatry* 49 (June 1992), pp. 488–492.

Einstein, Albert, and Leopold Infeld, *The Evolution of Physics* (New York: Simon & Schuster, 1966), 302 pp.

Eysenck, Hans, *Decline and Fall of the Freudian Empire* (New York: Penguin, 1985), 224 pp.

Fadiman, Clifton, ed., *Living Philosophies* (New York: Doubleday, 1990), 290 pp.

Farah, Martha, and James McClelland, "Neural Network Models and Cognitive Neuropsychology," *Psychiatric Annals* 22:3 (March 1922), pp. 148–153.

Fawcett, Jan, "Utilization Management—We Don't Have to Love It—We've Got to Learn About It," *Psychiatric Annals* 22:7 (July 1992), p. 354.

Feynman, Richard, *The Character of Physical Law* (Cambridge: MIT Press, 1965), 173 pp.

Finn, Chester, "The Campus: 'An Island of Repression in a Sea of Freedom,'" *Commentary* (September 1989), pp. 17–23.

Flanagan, Owen, *The Science of Mind* (Cambridge: MIT Press, 1991), 424 pp.

Flew, Anthony, ed., *Body, Mind, and Death* (New York: Macmillan, 1964), 306 pp.

Flew, Anthony, *A Dictionary of Philosophy* (New York: St. Martin's Press, 1979), 380 pp.

Fodor, Jerry, "The Mind–Body Problem," *Scientific American* 244 (January 1981), pp. 114–123.

Forward, Robert, "Spinning New Realities," *Science 80* 1 (December 1980), pp. 40–49.

Foucault, Michel, *Mental Illness and Psychology* (Berkeley: University of California Press, 1987), 90 pp.

Frankl, Viktor, *The Doctor and the Soul* (New York: Vintage, 1986), 318 pp.

Franklin, Jon, *Molecules of the Mind* (New York: Dell, 1987), 301 pp.

Frattaroli, Elio, "The Mind–Body Problem and the Choice of Intervention," *The Psychiatric Times* (November 1991), pp. 73–77.

Freedman, Daniel X., "The Search: Body, Mind, and Human Purpose," *American Journal of Psychiatry* 149:7 (July 1992), pp. 858–866.

Freedman, Daniel Z., and Peter van Nieuwenhuizen, "Supergravity and the Unification of the Laws of Physics," *Scientific American* 238 (February 1978), pp. 126–143.

Freeman, Walter, "The Physiology of Perception," *Scientific American* 264 (February 1991), pp. 78–85.

Freud, Sigmund, *An Autobiographical Study*, trans. James Strachey (New York: Norton, 1963), 126 pp.

Freud, Sigmund, *Beyond the Pleasure Principle*, trans. James Strachey (New York: Norton, 1961), 68 pp.

Freud, Sigmund, *An Outline of Psychoanalysis*, trans. James Strachey (New York: Norton, 1969), 75 pp.

Fromm, Erich, *The Sane Society* (New York: Henry Holt, 1955), 370 pp.

Gabbard, Glen, "Psychodynamic Psychiatry in the 'Decade of the Brain,'" *American Journal of Psychiatry* 149:8 (August 1992), pp. 991–998.

Gabbard, Glen, Susan Lazar, and Elizabeth Hersh, "Cost-Offset Studies Show Value of Psychotherapy," *Psychiatric Times* (August 1993), p. 21.

Gale, George, "The Anthropic Principle," *Scientific American* 245 (December 1981), pp. 154–171.

Gardner, Martin, *The Ambidextrous Universe* (New York: Scribner, 1979), 293 pp.

Gardner, Martin, "WAP, SAP, PAP & FAP: The Anthropic Cosmological Principle," *New York Review of Books* (8 May 1986), pp. 22–25.

Gardner, Martin, *The Whys of a Philosophical Scrivener* (New York: Quill, 1983), 453 pp.

Gazzaniga, Michael, *The Social Brain* (New York: Basic Books, 1985), 219 pp.

Gelernter, David, "The Metamorphosis of Information Management," *Scientific American* 261 (August 1989), pp. 66–73.

Gelman, David, Debra Rosenberg, Paul Kandell, and Rebecca Crandall, "Is the Mind an Illusion?" *Newsweek* (20 April 1992), pp. 71–72.

"Genes, Viruses, Hormones and Schizophrenia Etiology," *Clinical Psychiatry News* (August 1992), p. 22.

Genova, Paul, "Is American Psychiatry Terminally Ill?" *Psychiatric Times* (June 1993), pp. 19–20.

Georgi, Howard, "A Unified Theory of Elementary Particles and Forces," *Scientific American* 244 (April 1981), pp. 48–63.

Gibbins, Peter, *Particles and Paradoxes* (Cambridge: Cambridge University Press, 1987), 181 pp.

Gjertsen, Derek, *Science and Philosophy* (London: Penguin, 1989), 296 pp.

Glazer, William, "Overview of Utilization Management," *Psychiatric Annals* 22:7 (July 1992), p. 355.

Glazer, William, "Psychiatry and Medical Necessity," *Psychiatric Annals* 22:7 (July 1992), pp. 362–366.

Goldman, Harvey, *Max Weber and Thomas Mann* (Berkeley: University of California Press, 1988), 284 pp.

Goode, Erica, and Betsy Wagner, "Does Psychotherapy Work?" *US News and World Report* (24 May 1993), pp. 56–65.

Goodman, Aviel, "Organic Unity Theory: The Mind–Body Problem Revisited," *American Journal of Psychiatry* 148:5 (May 1991), pp. 553–563.

Goodwin, Donald, and Samuel Guze, *Psychiatric Diagnosis* (Oxford: Oxford University Press, 1984), 292 pp.

Gorman, David, and Jurgen Unutzer, "Brodmann's 'Missing' Numbers," *Neurology* 43 (January 1993), pp. 226–227.

Gould, Steven Jay, *Ever Since Darwin* (New York: Norton, 1977), 285 pp.

Green, Joseph, ed., *Borderland between Neurology and Psychiatry*, *Neurology Clinics* 2:1 (Philadelphia: Saunders, February 1984), 175 pp.

Green, Michael, "Superstrings," *Scientific American* 255:3 (September 1986), pp. 48–60.

Greenberg, Jay, and Stephen Mitchell, *Object Relations in Psychoanalytic Theory* (Cambridge: Harvard University Press, 1983), 436 pp.

Gregory, Richard, ed., *The Oxford Companion to the Mind* (Oxford: Oxford University Press, 1987), 856 pp.

Grob, Gerald, "Origins of DSM-I: A Study in Appearance and

Reality," *American Journal of Psychiatry* 148:4 (April 1991), pp. 421–431.

Gur, Ruben, Roland Erwin, and Raquel Gur, "Neurobehavioral Probes for Physiologic Neuroimaging Studies," *Archives of General Psychiatry* 49 (May 1992), pp. 409–414.

Hackett, Thomas, and Ned Cassem, *Massachusetts General Hospital Handbook of General Hospital Psychiatry* (Littleton: P. S. G., 1987), 658 pp.

Hales, Robert, and Stuart Yudofsky, eds., *Textbook of Neuropsychiatry* (Washington, DC, American Psychiatric Press, 1987), 490 pp.

Hampden-Turner, Charles, *Maps of the Mind* (New York: Collier Books, 1982), 224 pp.

Harper, Charlie, *Introduction to Mathematical Physics* (Englewood Cliffs, NJ: Prentice Hall, 1976), 301 pp.

Harvard Medical School Department of Continuing Education, *Psychiatry: A Comprehensive Review and Update*, syllabus for a course given 6–11 March, 1989.

Havel, Vaclav, "The End of the Modern Era," *The New York Times* (1 March 1992), p. E15.

Hawking, Stephen, *A Brief History of Time* (New York: Bantam Books, 1988), 198 pp.

Hearnshaw, L. S., *The Shaping of Modern Psychology* (London: Routledge, 1987), 423 pp.

Heilbroner, Robert, *Marxism: For and Against* (New York: Norton, 1980), 186 pp.

Heilbroner, Robert, *The Wordly Philosophers* (New York: Simon & Schuster, 1972), 347 pp.

Heilman, Kenneth, and Edward Valenstein, *Clinical Neuropsychology* (Oxford: Oxford University Press, 1985), 540 pp.

Heilman, Kenneth, Robert Watson, and Melvin Greer, *Handbook for Differential Diagnosis of Neurological Signs and Symptoms* (New York: Appleton-Century-Crofts, 1977), 231 pp.

Heinlein, Robert, *The Moon Is a Harsh Mistress* (New York: Ace, 1966), 302 pp.

Heisenberg, Werner, *Physics and Philosophy* (New York: Harper & Row, 1958), 213 pp.

Held, Donald, *Introduction to Critical Theory* (Berkeley: University of California Press, 1980), 511 pp.

Hendren, Robert, and Janet Hodde-Vargas, "Neuroimaging in Schizophrenia," *Psychiatric Times* (September 1992), pp. 17–21.

Hillman, James, *Emotion* (Evanston, IL: Northwestern University Press, 1962), 318 pp.

Himmelstein, David, and Steffie Woolhandler, "Clinton Plan Will Restrict Health Care Choice," *The New York Times* (26 September 1993), p. E14.

Hobson, J. Alan, *The Dreaming Brain* (New York: Basic Books, 1988), 319 pp.

Hoffman, Banesh, *The Strange Story of the Quantum* (New York: Dover, 1959), 285 pp.

Hoffman, Ralph, "Attractor Neural Networks and Psychotic Disorders," *Psychiatric Annals* 22:3 (March 1992), pp. 119–124.

Hofstadter, Douglas, *Gödel, Escher, Bach: An Eternal Golden Braid* (New York: Vintage, 1979), 777 pp.

Horgan, John, "Eugenics Revisited," *Scientific American* 268 (June 1993), p. 122–131.

Howard, Jonathan, *Darwin* (New York: Hill & Wang, 1982), 101 pp.

Hubben, William, *Dostoevsky, Kierkegaard, Nietzsche, and Kafka* (New York: Macmillan, 1952), 181 pp.

Hubel, David, "The Brain," in *The Brain*, eds. Gerard Piel *et al.* (San Francisco, W. H. Freeman, 1979), pp. 2–11.

Hughes, R. I. G., "Quantum Logic," *Scientific American* 245 (October 1981), pp. 202–213.

Hutchinson, G. E., "Man Talking or Thinking," *American Scientist* 64 (January–February 1976), pp. 22–27.

Huxley, Aldous, *Brave New Word/Brave New World Revisited* (New York: Harper & Row, 1960), 97 pp.

Innis, Robert, "Neuroreceptor Imaging With SPECT," *Journal of Clinical Psychiatry* 53:11 (November 1992 supplement), pp. 29–34.

Jacob, Francois, *The Logic of Life* (New York: Pantheon, 1973), 348 pp.

Jacob, Francois, *The Possible and the Actual* (New York: Pantheon, 1982), 70 pp.

Jaki, Stanley, *Brain, Mind and Computers* (South Bend, IN: Gateway, 1969), 267 pp.

Jeans, James, *Physics and Philosophy* (New York: Dover, 1981), 222 pp.

Johnson-Laird, Phillip N., *The Computer and the Mind* (Cambridge: Harvard University Press, 1988), 444 pp.

Jurgens, Hartmut, Heinz-Otto Peitgen, and Dietmar Saupe, "The Language of Fractals," *Scientific American* 263 (August 1990), pp. 60–67.

Kac, Mark, "Probability," *Scientific American* 211 (September 1964), pp. 92–96.

Kamin, Janet, "When Managed Care Manages Psychotherapy," *The New York Times* (13 May 1993), p. A22.

Kandel, Eric, "Psychotherapy and the Single Synapse," *New England Journal of Medicine* 301:19 (8 November 1979), pp. 1028–1037.

Kandel, Eric, and James Schwartz, eds., *Principles of Neural Science* (New York: Elsevier, 1981), 731 pp.

Kaplan, Harold, and Benjamin Sadock, *Synopsis of Psychiatry* (Baltimore: Williams & Wilkins, 1988), 725 pp.

Karel, Richard, "Congress Gets Earful on Psych Hospitals," *The Psychiatric News* (19 June 1992), pp. 1, 26.

Katz, Bernard, *Nerve, Muscle and Synapse* (New York: McGraw-Hill, 1966), 193 pp.

Kauffman, Stuart, "Antichaos and Adaptation," *Scientific American* 265 (August 1991), pp. 78–84.

Kerner, George, *Three Philosophical Moralists* (Oxford: Clarendon, 1990), 204 pp.

Kessen, William, and Emily Cahan, "A Century of Psychology: From Subject to Object to Agent," *American Scientist* 24 (November–December 1986), pp. 640–649.

Klass, Donald, and David Daly, eds., *Current Practice of Clinical Electroencephalography* (New York: Raven, 1979), 532 pp.

Kline, Morris, *Mathematics, the Loss of Certainty* (New York: Oxford University Press, 1980), 366 pp.

Koestler, Arthur, *The Ghost in the Machine* (London: Penguin, 1967), 384 pp.

Kolata, Gina, "Does Gödel's Theorem Matter to Mathematics?," *Science* 218:19 (November 1982), pp. 779–780.

Kolata, Gina, "Improved Scanner Watches the Brain as It Thinks," *The New York Times* (14 July 1992), pp. C1, C6.

Kramer, Edna, *The Nature and Growth of Modern Mathematics* (Princeton: Princeton University Press, 1981), 758 pp.

Krupnick, Janice, and Harold Alan Pincus, "The Cost-Effectiveness of Psychotherapy: A Plan for Research," *American Journal of Psychiatry* 149:10 (October 1992), pp. 1295–1305.

Kuper, Adam, and Jessica Kuper, eds., *The Social Science Encyclopedia* (New York: Routledge, 1985), 916 pp.

Ladd, Scott, *The Computer and the Brain* (New York: Bantam, 1986), 186 pp.

Lasch, Christopher, *The Culture of Narcissism* (New York: Warner Books, 1979), 447 pp.

Lasch, Christopher, *The Minimal Self* (New York: Norton, 1984), 317 pp.

Lauerman, John, "Windows on the Brain: Functional Brain Imaging Techniques Add Objective Scale to Psychiatric Evaluation and Treatment," *Psychiatric Times* (February 1993), pp. 16–17.

Lederman, Leon, "Science and the Bottom Line," *The New York Times* (16 September 1993), p. A23.

Le Doux, Joseph, and Williams Hirst, eds., *Mind and Brain* (Cambridge: Cambridge University Press, 1986), 449 pp.

Lee, Seungho Howard, and Krishna, C. V. G. Rao, *Cranial Computed Tomography and M. R. I.* (New York: McGraw-Hill, 1987), 858 pp.

Leith, Emmett N., and Juris Upatnieks, "Photography by Laser," *Scientific American* 212 (June 1965), pp. 24–35.

Lessing, Doris, "Language and the Lunatic Fringe," *The New York Times* (26 June 1992), p. A27.

Lezak, Muriel, *Neuropsychological Assessment* (Oxford: Oxford University Press 1983), 768 pp.

Liberman, Robert P., and Patrick W. Corrigan, "Is Schizophrenia a Neurological Disorder?" *Journal of Neuropsychiatry* 4:2 (Spring 1992), pp. 119–124.

Li, David, and David Spiegel, "A Neural Network Model of Dissociative Disorders," *Psychiatric Annals* 22:3 (March 1922), pp. 144–147.

Lidz, Theodore, "Images in Psychiatry: Adolf Meyer," *American Journal of Psychiatry* 150:7 (July 1993), p. 1098.

Lieberson, Jonathan, "The 'Truth' of Karl Popper," *New York Review of Books* (18 November 1982), pp. 67–68.

Lindsay, Robert Bruce, and Henry Margenau, *Foundations of Physics* (Woodbridge, NJ: Oxbow Press, 1981), 542 pp.

Linnoila, Markku, and Matti Virkkunen, "Aggression, Suicidality, and Serotonin," *Journal of Clinical Psychiatry* 53:10 (October 1992 supplement), pp. 46–51.

Lishman, W. A., *Organic Psychiatry* (Oxford: Blackwell, 1987), 745 pp.

Lockwood, Michael, *Mind, Brain and the Quantum* (Oxford: Basil Blackwood, 1989), 365 pp.

Longair, M. S., *Theoretical Concepts in Physics* (Cambridge: Cambridge University Press, 1984), 366 pp.

Losee, John, *A Historical Introduction to the Philosophy of Science* (New York: Oxford University Press, 1980), 248 pp.

Lund, R. D., *Development and Plasticity of the Brain* (New York: Oxford University Press, 1978), 370 pp.

Luria, A. R., *The Making of Mind*, eds. Michael Cole and Shiela Cole (Cambridge: Harvard University Press, 1979), 234 pp.

Luria, A. R., *The Working Brain*, trans. Basil Haigh (New York: Basic Books, 1973), 398 pp.

MacIntyre, Alasdair, *A Short History of Ethics* (New York: Macmillan, 1966), 280 pp.

MacLane, Saunders, "Mathematical Models of Space," *American Scientist* 68 (March 1980), pp. 184–191.

Madore, Barry, and Wendy Freedman, "Self-organizing Structures," *American Scientist* 75 (May–June 1987), pp. 252–259.

Manin, Y. I., *Mathematics and Physics* (Boston: Birkauser, 1981), 99 pp.

Mann, Charles, "How Many Is Too Many?" *Atlantic Monthly* (February 1993), pp. 47–67.

Marcel, Gabriel, *The Philosophy of Existentialism* (New York: Citadel, 1984), 128 pp.

Marcus, Eric, *Psychosis and Near Psychosis* (New York: Springer-Verlag, 1992), 308 pp.

Marcuse, Herbert, *Eros and Civilization* (Boston: Beacon Press, 1966), 277 pp.

Marcuse, Herbert, *Negations* (London: Free Association Books, 1988), 290 pp.

Marcuse, Herbert, *One-Dimensional Man* (Boston: Beacon Press, 1964), 260 pp.

Margenau, Henry, *The Nature of Physical Reality* (Woodbridge, NJ: Oxbow Press, 1977), 479 pp.

Marsh, Ken, *The Way the New Technology Works* (New York: Simon & Schuster, 1982), 240 pp.

May, Rollo, *The Courage to Create* (New York: Bantam, 1975), 173 pp.

McGeer, Patrick, John Eccles, and Edith McGeer, *Molecular Biology of the Mammalian Brain* (New York: Plenum, 1978), 644 pp.

"Measuring Psychiatry's Cost-Effectiveness: When a Dollar Saved Is Not a Dollar Earned," *Psychiatric News* (19 June 1992), p. 24.

Medawar, Peter, *Pluto's Republic* (Oxford: Oxford University Press, 1982), 351 pp.

Mender, Donald, notes for a lecture on CT, MRI, and PET scanning in psychiatry given in 1988 at St. John's Episcopal Hospital, Smithtown, New York.

Mender, Donald, notes for a seminar on Soviet psychiatric diagnosis given in 1987 at the Payne Whitney Clinic, New York, New York.

Merriam, Arnold, Alice A. Medalia, and Bernard Wyszynski, "Schizophrenia as a Neurobehavioral Disorder," *Psychiatric Annals* 23:4 (April 1993), pp. 171–178.

Mesulam, M. Marsel, ed., *Principles of Behavioral Neurology* (Philadelphia: F. A. Davis, 1985), 405 pp.

Miller, David, ed., *Popper Selections* (Princeton: Princeton University Press, 1985), 479 pp.

Miller, Glenn, "Insanity Standards," *Psychiatric Annals* 22: 12 (December 1992), pp. 626–631.

Monod, Jacques, *Chance and Necessity* (New York: Vintage, 1971), 199 pp.

Moore, Daniel, "Utilization Management and Outpatient Treatment," *Psychiatric Annals* 22:7 (July 1992), pp. 373–377.

Morisa, John, *Brain Imaging in Psychiatry* (Washington: American Psychiatric Press, 1984), 93 pp.

Morowitz, Harold, *Cosmic Joy and Local Pain* (New York: Scribner, 1987), 321 pp.

Morowitz, Harold, *Mayonnaise and the Origin of Life* (New York: Berkeley, 1985), 244 pp.

Morowitz, Harold, *The Wine of Life* (New York: Bantam, 1979), 227 pp.

Motz, Lloyd, and Jefferson Hane Weaver, *The Concepts of Science* (New York: Plenum, 1993), 435 pp.

Motz, Lloyd, and Jefferson Hane Weaver, *The Story of Mathematics* (New York: Plenum, 1988), 356 pp.

Mountcastle, Vernon, ed., *Medical Physiology*, Volume 1 (St. Louis: Mosby, 1980), p. iii.

Mundt, Christoph, "Images in Psychiatry: Karl Jaspers," *American Journal of Psychiatry* 150:8 (August 1993), pp. 1244–1245.

Nagel, Ernest and James R. Newman, *Gödel's Proof* (New York: New York University Press, 1958), 118 pp.

Nambu, Yoichiro, "The Confinement of Quarks," *Scientific American* 235 (November 1976), pp. 48–60.

Nehamas, Alexander, "Subject and Abject," *The New Republic* (15 February 1993), pp. 27–36.

Neu, Jerome, ed., *The Cambridge Companion to Freud* (Cambridge: Cambridge University Press, 1991), 356 pp.

Nicholi, Armand, ed., *The New Harvard Guide to Psychiatry* (Cambridge: Bellknap Press, 1988), 865 pp.

Norman, Donald, *Memory and Attention* (New York: Wiley, 1969), 201 pp.

Oldroyd, David, *The Arch of Knowledge* (New York: Methuen, 1986), 413 pp.

Ortega y Gasset, José, *The Revolt of the Masses*, authorized anonymous translation from the Spanish (New York: Norton, 1932), 204 pp.

Orwell, George, *1984* (New York: Signet, 1961), 267 pp.

Pagels, Heinz, *The Dreams of Reason* (New York: Bantam, 1988), 352 pp.

Paglia, Camille, "Ninnies, Pedants, Tyrants and Other Academics," *The New York Times Book Review* (5 May 1991), pp. C3, C29, C33.

Pais, Abraham, *Subtle Is the Lord* (Oxford: Oxford University Press, 1982), 552 pp.

Palmer, Donald, *Does the Center Hold?* (Mountain View, CA: Mayfield, 1991), 529 pp.

Palmer, Donald, *Looking at Philosophy* (Mountain View, CA: Mayfield, 1988), 401 pp.

Papke, C. Owen, *The Evolution of Progress* (New York: Random House, 1993), 382 pp.

Parker, Barry, *Search for a Supertheory* (New York: Plenum, 1987), 292 pp.

Paulos, John Allen, "Fearful Symmetry," *The New York Times Book Review* (28 June 1992), p. 11.

Peat, F. David, *Superstrings and the Search for the Theory of Everything* (Chicago: Contemporary Books, 1988), 362 pp.

Penrose, Roger, *The Emperor's New Mind* (Oxford: Oxford University Press, 1989), 466 pp.

Piel, Gerard, *et al.*, eds., *The Brain* (San Francisco: W. H. Freeman, 1979), 149 pp.

Pierce, Calvin, "APA Ready to Launch Practice Guidelines Era," *Clinical Psychiatry News* 20:6 (June 1992), pp. 1, 22.

Pincus, Harold Alan, and Theodora Fine, "The 'Anatomy' of Research Funding of Mental Illness and Addictive Disorders," *Archives of General Psychiatry* 49 (July 1992), pp. 573–579.

Pincus, Jonathan, and Gary Tucker, *Behavioral Neurology* (Oxford: Oxford University Press, 1985), 322 pp.

Pollack, John, *Technical Methods in Philosophy* (Boulder, CO: Westview, 1990), 126 pp.

Popper, Karl, *Unended Quest* (Glasgow: Collins, 1976), 270 pp.

Powers, Jonathan, *Philosophy and the New Physics* (New York: Methuen, 1982), 203 pp.

Pribram, Karl, "The Neurophysiology of Remembering," *Scientific American* 220 (January 1969), pp. 73–86.

Priest, Stephen, *Theories of the Mind* (Boston: Houghton Mifflin, 1991), 233 pp.

Prigogine, Ilya, and Isabella Stengers, *Order Out of Chaos* (New York: Bantam, 1982), 349 pp.

"Psychotherapy Under the Knife," *U.S. News and World Report* (24 May 1993), p. 64.

Reichenbach, Hans, *The Rise of Scientific Philosophy* (Berkeley: University of California Press, 1951), 333 pp.

Relman, Arnold, "What Market Values Are Doing to Medicine," *Atlantic Monthly* (March 1992), pp. 99–106.

Restak, Richard, "Brain by Design," *The Sciences* (September–October 1993), pp. 27–33.

Restak, Richard, "See No Evil," *The Sciences* (July–August 1992), pp. 16–21.

Rieff, Philip, *Freud: The Mind of the Moralist* (Chicago: University of Chicago Press, 1979), 440 pp.

Rosensweig, Mark, and Edward Bennett, eds., *Neural Mechanisms of Memory and Learning* (Cambridge: MIT Press, 1976), 636 pp.

Rosenthal, Elisabeth, "Insurers Second-Guess Doctors, Provoking Debate over Savings," *The New York Times* (24 January 1993), p. 1, 22.

Ross, G. MacDonald, *Leibnitz* (Oxford: Oxford University Press, 1984), 121 pp.

Rothman, Tony, "The Short Life of Evariste Galois," *Scientific American* 246 (April 1982), pp. 136–149.

Rowland, Lewis, P., ed., *Merritt's Textbook of Neurology* (Philadelphia: Lea & Febiger, 1984), 774 pp.

Rucker, Rudy, *Infinity and the Mind* (New York: Bantam, 1982), 366 pp.

Rucker, Rudy, *Mind Tools* (Boston: Houghton Mifflin, 1987), 328 pp.

Russell, Bertrand, *A History of Western Philosophy* (New York: Simon & Schuster, 1945), 590 pp.

Sarnat, Harvey, and Martin Netsky, *Evolution of the Nervous System* (New York: Oxford University Press, 1974), 318 pp.

Sartre, Jean-Paul, *The Transcendence of the Ego* (New York: Hill & Wang, 1992), 119 pp.

Sawyer, W. W., *A Concrete Approach to Abstract Algebra* (New York: Dover, 1959), 234 pp.

Schatzberg, Alan, and Jonathan Cole, *Manual of Clinical Psychopharmacology* (Washington: American Psychiatric Press, 1986), 294 pp.

Schellenberg, James, *Masters of Social Psychology* (New York: Oxford University Press, 1978), 141 pp.

Schilpp, Paul Arthur, ed., *Albert Einstein: Philosopher-Scientist*, Volume 7, *Library of Living Philosophers* (London: Cambridge University Press, 1970), 781 pp.

Schrödinger, Erwin, *My View of the World* (Woodbridge, NJ: Ox Bow Press, 1983), 110 pp.

Schrödinger, Erwin, *What Is Life?/Mind and Matter* (Cambridge: Cambridge University Press, 1967), 178 pp.

Schröeder, Manfred, *Fractals, Chaos, Power Laws* (New York: W. H. Freeman, 1991), 429 pp.

Schuckit, Marc, "An Introduction and Overview to Clinical Applications of Neuro SPECT in Psychiatry," *Journal of Clinical Psychiatry* 53:11 (November 1992 supplement), pp. 3–6.

Schutz, Bernard, *Geometrical Methods of Mathematical Physics* (Cambridge: Cambridge University Press, 1980), 250 pp.

Scruton, Roger, *From Descartes to Wittgenstein* (New York: Harper & Row, 1981), 298 pp.

Scruton, Roger, *Kant* (Oxford: Oxford University Press, 1982), 99 pp.

Searle, John, "Is the Brain's Mind a Computer Program?" *Scientific American* 262 (January 1990), pp. 26–31.

Searle, John, *Minds, Brains and Science* (Cambridge: Harvard University Press, 1984), 107 pp.

Searle, John, *The Rediscovery of the Mind* (Cambridge: MIT Press, 1992), 270 pp.

Selkirk, Errol, *Computers for Beginners* (New York: Writers and Readers Publishing, 1988), 187 pp.

Servan-Schreiber, David, and Jonathan Cohen, "A Neural Network Model of Catecholamine Modulation of Behavior," *Psychiatric Annals* 22:3 (March 1922), pp. 125–130.

Shader, Richard, ed., *Manual of Psychiatric Therapeutics* (Boston: Little Brown, 1975), 362 pp.

Shapiro, Stuart, and Saul Teukolsky, "Black Holes, Naked Singularities and Cosmic Censorship," *American Scientist* 79 (July– August 1991), pp. 330–343.

Sherman, Carl, "MDs Urged to Take Lead Role in Efforts to Reduce Violence," *Clinical Psychiatry News* (January 1993), p. 23.

Shumway, David, *Michel Foucault* (Charlottesville: University Press of Virginia, 1989), 178 pp.

Siever, Larry J., and Kenneth L. Davis, "A Psychobiological Perspective on the Personality Disorders," *American Journal of Psychiatry* 148:12 (December 1991), pp. 1647–1658.

Singer, Peter, *Hegel* (Oxford: Oxford University Press, 1983), 97 pp.

Singer, Peter, *Marx* (Oxford: Oxford University Press, 1980), 82 pp.

Singh, Janjit, *Great Ideas of Modern Mathematics* (New York: Dover, 1959), 312 pp.

Skinner, Quentin, ed., *The Return of Grand Theory in the Human Sciences* (Cambridge: Cambridge University Press, 1985), 214 pp.

Sklar, Lawrence, *Space, Time, and Spacetime* (Berkeley: University of California Press, 1976), 422 pp.

Slatkin, Stephen, "Short-Term Treatment, Better Results: IS-TDP," *Psychiatric Times* (March 1993), pp. 23–27.

Smith, Huston, *The Religions of Man* (New York: Harper & Row, 1986), pp. 18–120.

Smith, John Maynard, "The Evolution of Behavior," *Scientific American* 236 (September 1978), 509 pp.

Solomon, Robert, *Continental Philosophy Since 1750* (Oxford: Oxford University Press, 1988), 214 pp.

Sondheimer, Ernst, and Alan Rogerson, *Numbers and Infinity* (Cambridge: Cambridge University Press, 1981), 172 pp.

Spergel, David, and Neil Turok, "Textures and Cosmic Structure," *Scientific American* 266 (March 1992), pp. 52–59.

Spitzer, Robert L., Michael B. First, Janet B. W. Williams, Kenneth Kendler, Harold Alan Pincus, and Gary Tucker, "Now Is the Time to Retire the Term 'Organic Mental Disorder,'" *American Journal of Psychiatry* 149:2 (February 1992), pp. 240–244.

Steen, Lynn Arthur, "New Models of the Real Number Line," *Scientific American* 255 (August 1971), pp. 92–99.

Steen, Lynn Arthur, ed., *Mathematics Today* (New York: Random House, 1978), 367 pp.

Stoudemire, Alan, and Barry Fogel, eds., *Principles of Medical Psychiatry* (Orlando, FL: Grune and Stratton, 1987), 719 pp.

Sutton, Jeffrey, Adam Mamelak, and J. Allan Hobson, "Modeling States of Waking and Sleeping," *Psychiatric Annals* 22:3 (March 1992), pp. 137–143.

Szasz, Thomas, *The Myth of Mental Illness* (New York: Harper & Row, 1974), 297 pp.

Tardiff, Kenneth, "The Current State of Psychiatry in the Treatment of Violent Patients," *Archives of General Psychiatry* 49 (June 1992), pp. 493–499.

Tarnas, Richard, *The Passion of the Western Mind* (New York: Crown, 1981), 543 pp.

Teichman, Jenny, *Philosophy and the Mind* (Oxford: Basil Blackwell, 1988), 136 pp.

Teller, Edward, *The Pursuit of Simplicity* (Malibu: Pepperdine University Press, 1980), 173 pp.

Teresi, Dick, "Perhaps This Universe Is Only a Test," *The New York Times Book Review* (5 September 1993), p. 11.

t'Hooft, Gerard, "Gauge Theories of the Forces between Elementary Particles," *Scientific American* 242 (June 1980), pp. 104–138.

Thorne, J. O., ed., *Chambers's Biographical Dictionary* (New York: St. Martin's Press, 1962), 1432 pp.

Tillich, Paul, *The Courage To Be* (New Haven: Yale University Press, 1980), 197 pp.

Tomb, David, *Psychiatry for the House Officer* (Baltimore: Williams & Wilkins, 1988), 236 pp.

Tucker, Miriam, "Clozapine-like Antipsychotics Seen as Wave of the Future," *Clinical Psychiatric News* (January 1993), pp. 1, 13.

Tucker, Robert, *Philosophy and Myth in Karl Marx* (London: Cambridge University Press, 1972), 263 pp.

Van Heertum, Ronald, "Brain SPECT Imaging and Psychiatry," *Journal of Clinical Psychiatry* 53:11 (November 1992 supplement), pp. 7–12.

Varmus, Harold, and Marc Kirschner, "Don't Undermine Basic Research," *The New York Times* (29 September 1992), p. A27.

Volkow, Nora, D., and Laurence R. Tancredi, "Biological Correlates of Mental Activity Studied With PET," *American Journal of Psychiatry* 148:4 (April 1991), pp. 439–443.

Volkow, Nora, and Laurence Tancredi, "Current and Future Applications of SPECT in Clinical Psychiatry," *Journal of Clinical Psychiatry* 53:11 (November 1992 supplement), pp. 26–28.

Von Neumann, John, *The Computer and the Brain* (New Haven: Yale University Press, 1958), 822 pp.

Wallich, Paul, "Silicon Babies," *Scientific American* 265 (December 1991), pp. 124–134.

Walton, John, revising author, *Brain's Diseases of the Nervous System* (Oxford: Oxford University Press, 1977), 1277 pp.

Weinberg, Steven, *Dreams of a Final Theory* (New York: Pantheon Books, 1992), 334 pp.

Weinberg, Steven, "Unified Theories of Elementary-Particle Interaction," *Scientific American* 231 (July 1974), pp. 50–59.

Weinberger, Daniel, "A Connectionist Approach to the Prefrontal Cortex," *Journal of Neuropsychiatry* 5:3 (Summer 1993), pp. 241–253.

Weyl, Hermann, *Symmetry* (Princeton: Princeton University Press, 1952), 168 pp.

White, Morton, ed., *The Age of Analysis* (New York: Mentor, 1955), 253 pp.

Wigner, Eugene, *Symmetries and Reflections* (Woodbridge, NJ: Oxbow Press, 1979), 280 pp.

Wile, Lawrence, "Quantum Concepts," *Psychiatric Times* (February 1993), p. 9.

Williams, Bernard, "Leviathan's Program," *The New York Review of Books* (11 June 1987), pp. 33–35.

Wilson, Edward O., *On Human Nature* (New York: Bantam, 1978), 272 pp.

Wilson, Kenneth, "Problems in Physics with Many Scales of Length," *Scientific American* 241 (August 1979), pp. 158–179.

Wilson, Mitchell, "DSM-III and the Transformation of American Psychiatry: A History," *American Journal of Psychiatry* 150:3 (March 1993), pp. 399–410.

Winson, Jonathan, *Brain and Psyche* (Garden City, NY: Doubleday, 1985), 300 pp.

Witelson, Sandra, "Cognitive Neuroanatomy," *Neurology* 42 (April 1992), pp. 709–713.

Woods, Scott, "Regional Cerebral Blood Flow Imaging With SPECT in Psychiatric Disease: Focus on Schizophrenia, Anxiety Disorders, and Substance Abuse," *Journal of Clinical Psychiatry* 53:11 (November 1992 supplement), pp. 20–25.

Young, J. F., *Information Theory* (New York: Wiley, 1971), 168 pp.

Yudofsky, Stuart C., and Robert E. Hales, "The Reemergence of Neuropsychiatry: Definition and Direction," *Journal of Neuropsychiatry* 1:1 (Winter 1989), pp. 1–6.

Yudofsky, Stuart C., and Robert E. Hales, "When Patients Ask . . . What Is Neuropsychiatry?" *Journal of Neuropsychiatry* 1:4 (Fall 1989), pp. 362–365.

Index

Immune function, 24
Impulsive behavior, 22, 23, 25
Individual psychology, 160
Industrial Revolution, 135
Inhibitory synapses, 63, 78
Inquiry into the Nature and Causes of the Wealth of Nations, An (Smith), 134
Insanity defense, 150
Insight-oriented psychotherapy, 28, 171
Institute for New Generation Computer Technology, 125
Institute of Social Research, 141
Insulin tolerance test, 22
Insulin treatment, 13
Integers, 49, 83
Integrative Action of the Nervous System, The (Sherrington), 61
Intentionality, 94–100, 115, 117
   computer metaphors and, 94, 96–100
   as curvature, 108
   gauge fields and, 113
   in psychoanalysis, 157, 161, 162, 169, 170, 171–172
International Congress of Psychology, 125
International Psychoanalytic Association, 159
Interpretation of Dreams, The (Freud), 154
Intersubjectivity, 124, 125
Introduction to Comparative Anatomy, An (Morgan), 66
Introduction to Mathematical Philosophy (Russell), 50
Intuitionism, 51–52
Invariance, 59, 106–107, 108
   global, 106–107, 108, 116, 131
   local, 106, 109, 115, 131, 132
   parity, 43
   rotational, 43, 105
Invariant principle, 43–44

Invariant substance, 44, 51
Iproniazid, 15

Jackson, John Hughlings, 66–67, 155
Jacob, Francois, 162–163
James, Henry, Jr., 160
James, Henry, Sr., 160
James, William, 160–161, 163
Jaspers, Karl, 164–165
Joan of Arc, 5
Johnson-Laird, Phillip, 76, 82
Jokes and Their Relation to the Unconscious (Freud), 154
Journal of Social Research, 141
Judd, C. H., 125
Jung, Carl, 57, 154, 159–160
Jung's Word Association Test, 57
Just noticeable differences, law of, 55

Kandel, Eric, 2–4, 16, 169
Kant, Immanuel, 36–37, 39, 88, 106, 110, 119
Kepler, Johannes, 33, 101
Keynes, John Maynard, 136
Kierkegaard, Søren, 164
Klein, Felix, 42, 52, 106
Koestler, Arthur, 120
Koffka, Kurt, 104
Köhler, Wolfgang, 104
Kraepelin, Emil, 12, 164
Kronecker, Leopold, 52
Kuhn, Roland, 15
Kuhn, Thomas, 89

Labor, 140–141
   division of, 134, 144, 149
Laborit, Henri, 14
Labor theory of value, 144
Labour Party (Britain), 135
Laing, R. D., 164
Language
   brain damage and, 69
   collective self-alienation and, 121–122